MW00850399

PRAISE FOR

Can Fasting Save Your Life?

If you are bewildered by the varieties of fasting, read Dr. Myers's and Dr. Goldhamer's *Can Fasting Save* Your *Life?* Theirs are the voices of pioneering experts with unsurpassed encyclopedic knowledge in this emerging life-saving discipline.

Caldwell B. Esselstyn Jr., MD
Author of *Prevent and Reverse Heart Disease*

Fasting is an important tool to facilitate healing and recovery and has many important therapeutic applications, yet it is often completely ignored by physicians, limiting their ability as healers. This book can bring the olden art of fasting (and the practice of eating a healthful diet) into modern healthcare where it belongs.

Joel Fuhrman, MD
Author of seven New York Times bestsellers, including *Eat for Life*

This is the definitive guide about fasting, the science behind it, and how to do it right. This powerful approach to health has given new tools to physicians and has been life-changing for countless individuals. Drawing on decades of experience and careful study, Drs. Myers and Goldhamer have provided everything you need to know to put that power to work.

Neal D. Barnard, MD, FACC
Adjunct professor, George Washington University School of Medicine
President of Physicians Committee for Responsible Medicine

Can Fasting Save Your *Life?* is the best fasting book available, offering clinical insights and a clarion call to the research community to study this neglected lifestyle intervention.

Michael Greger, MD
Author of *How Not to Die* and founder of nutritionfacts.org

The best and last hope I have been able to offer my patients over the past 40 years is a water fast under the direction of Dr. Alan Goldhamer. Water is the ultimate no-fat, low-cholesterol treatment that every person should try before declaring defeat.

John McDougall, MD
Founder of the McDougall Program

I have personally experienced the remarkable effects of water-only fasting at TrueNorth Health Center. I have seen the benefits for friends and family members that I have referred for fasting. The clinical outcomes seem to defy explanations, yet this new book provides valuable insights into the proposed mechanisms and physiological changes that are facilitated by fasting.

This book is a valuable resource for anyone interested in optimizing their health or in understanding the phenomenon of fasting. Adhering to the recommendations included in this book might just elevate and prolong the quality of your life.

Joseph Brimhall, DC
President of University of Western States

This book is unique in that it combines Dr. Alan Goldhamer's more than 40 years of clinical experience supervising fasting in more than 25,000 patients with Columbia University research scientist Dr. Toshia Meyers's ability to understand and communicate the science of fasting. If you are a researcher, a clinician, or an average person interested in reversing or preventing disease with fasting, the information in this book could save your life.

Rich Roll
Author of *Finding Ultra* and host of *The Rich Roll Podcast*

Fasting has captured the attention of the health conscious. No longer just the stuff of stories, fasting has cutting-edge research to back up its efficacy. In this book you will learn about the history, the anecdotes, and the 21st century science on fasting. You will learn from the world's foremost expert in the clinical application of fasting on just how powerful fasting really is and why it might just save your life.

Stephan Esser, MD
Author and motivational speaker; cofounder and director of Esser Health

It is long past time for the healing professions and the public to learn about, utilize, and benefit from the healing powers unleashed by water-only fasting, and *Can Fasting Save* Your *Life?* provides the needed guidance. It is an easy, informative read—and, yes, might even help save your life!

Michael Klaper, MD
Director of Moving Medicine Forward initiative

One of the more difficult truths to grasp is how doing nothing is often the best solution. Yet whether the problem is giving children a head start to supplement their education (a complete failure) or fluoridating a municipal water supply for some theoretical benefit (an enormously destructive practice), the drive to do something blinds otherwise capable people from seeing the truth. Here we have perhaps the most comprehensive case of this human error laid bare before our eyes.

Can Fasting Save Your *Life?* tells the story that for a huge plethora of health problems, doing nothing—intelligently—is often the very best move on the chessboard. This proposal is highly counterintuitive, yet it is true. Whether you are a physician or a layperson, this exceptional book provides a rare opportunity for clarity in how to optimize the healing process. Once you see how well fasting works, you will never look at health problems the same way.

Douglas Lisle, PhD
Coauthor of *The Pleasure Trap*

Drs. Myers and Goldhamer present a compelling argument in their new book, *Can Fasting Save* Your *Life?* Through scientific analysis and practical understanding, they demonstrate how water-only fasting, followed by a nutritious diet, can effectively reverse conditions like metabolic dysfunction, obesity, and hypertension.

This essential guide outlines the full potential of fasting as a tool for improving health and curing various ailments. If you're seeking concrete answers and a clear approach to better well-being, then reading *Can Fasting Save* Your *Life?* will give you a definitive answer. Spoiler alert: the answer is a resounding yes!

Jeff Nelson
Founder of VegSource Interactive

CAN FASTING SAVE YOUR LIFE?

TOSHIA MYERS, PhD

ALAN GOLDHAMER, DC

Healthy Living Publications

Summertown, Tennessee

Library of Congress Cataloging-in-Publication Data

Names: Myers, Toshia, 1977- author. | Goldhamer, Alan, author.
Title: Can fasting save your life? / Toshia Myers, PhD, Alan Goldhamer, DC.

Description: Summertown, Tennessee : Book Publishing Company, [2024] | Includes bibliographical references and index. | Summary: "Reports on classic and cutting-edge fasting research, concepts, and data, including clinical trials and case reports published by the TrueNorth Health Foundation in peer-reviewed journals. Further describes the capacity of fasting to reduce visceral fat, and to lower biomarkers of fatty liver, systemic inflammation, and insulin resistance, thereby allowing cells, tissues, and organs to recover from conditions that are conventionally considered unresolvable"— Provided by publisher.
Identifiers: LCCN 2023053170 (print) | LCCN 2023053171 (ebook) | ISBN 9781570674198 (hardback) | ISBN 9781570678196 (ebook)
Subjects: LCSH: Fasting—Therapeutic use. | Diet therapy.
Classification: LCC RM226 .M94 2024 (print) | LCC RM226 (ebook) | DDC 613.2/5—dc23/eng/20240125
LC record available at https://lccn.loc.gov/2023053170
LC ebook record available at https://lccn.loc.gov/2023053171

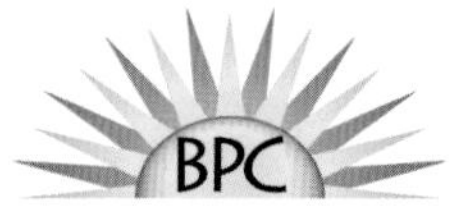

We chose to print this title on sustainably harvested paper stock certified by the Forest Stewardship Council, an independent auditor of responsible forestry practices. For more information, visit us.fsc.org.

Printed in the United States of America

Healthy Living Publications
A division of Book Publishing Company
PO Box 99
Summertown, TN 38483
888-260-8458
bookpubco.com

ISBN: 978-1-57067-419-8
eBook ISBN: 978-1-57067-819-6

29 28 27 26 25 24 1 2 3 4 5 6 7 8 9

Disclaimer: The information in this book is presented for educational purposes only. It is not intended to be a substitute for the medical advice of a physician, dietitian, or other health-care professional.

CONTENTS

Dedication

To the patients of the
TrueNorth Health Center

FOREWORD

Fasting, one of the oldest health remedies known to humankind, has not received the attention it deserves in the medical community. For almost 40 years, Dr. Goldhamer has operated his clinic at TrueNorth Health Center in Santa Rosa, California. His waiting list of patients is a testament to his success.

I can affirm the value of fasting, both personally and professionally. In the early 1990s, I incurred a neurological condition that affected my speech. It had actually begun 25 years earlier when I had heavy exposure to an exceptionally toxic chemical called chick edema factor,[1] which was subsequently given the name dioxin (of Vietnam Agent Orange fame). According to a Canadian government food and drug testing lab, my blood contained 800 times the maximum safe level that was later set for dioxin! I had tried virtually everything I could think of to resolve my problem but without success. So, in one final effort, I tried water-only fasting, which entailed two 14-day fasts, one year apart. Being a professional researcher and teaching toxicology, pharmacology, and nutrition, I was aware of evidence showing that fasting might clear the body of such toxins.

After the first fast, my blood level of the toxin dropped to "undetectable," according to a clinical lab test at UCLA, but I didn't have any improvement in my condition. However, I tried a second fast a year later, and my problem was fully resolved about a month afterward. I reasoned that although the level of dioxin in my blood disappeared after the first fast, it seemed to require an additional year for me to experience its clinical benefit. During that year, I read a report from France stating that dioxin causes demyelination (damage to the protective myelin sheath that surrounds nerve fibers in the brain, optic nerves, and spinal cord), which is considered a permanent condition. Nevertheless, I imagined that remyelination, similar to the revascularization of blood vessels, might be possible, especially when sustained by a whole-food plant-based diet (with minimal or no added salt,

[1] Campbell C, Friedman L. Chemical assay and isolation of chick edema factor in biological materials. *J Am Assoc Agri Chem* 1966; 49: 824-828.

sugar, or fat), which has worked so well for reversing chronic degenerative diseases. I believe that is what had actually happened.

On my second fast, I was joined by my wife, Karen, who had been diagnosed with advanced melanoma (stage 3, because of the presence of melanocytes in her lymph gland). She had refused the recommended surgical removal of the nearby lymph gland and chemotherapy in favor of a strict whole-food plant-based diet. She did a water-only 14-day fast and unexpectedly resolved a long-standing asthma condition in the process as well as all evidence of the advanced melanoma. This was nearly 18 years ago, and Karen has had no further problems with these conditions since then.

And there's more. My colleague at Cornell, Banoo Parpia, PhD, and I analyzed more than 170 patient records in the TrueNorth Health Center database to assess the effects of water-only fasting on blood pressure. The outcomes were remarkably impressive. The greater the blood pressure at the start, the larger the decrease, resulting in an almost perfectly linear regression to the healthiest level. These results were published in the peer-reviewed medical literature in collaboration with Dr. Goldhamer.[2]

There's still more. During my stays at TrueNorth Health Center, I became acquainted with many of Dr. Goldhamer's patients, who experienced a wide variety of ailments. Based on their narratives, I can say with great confidence that the benefits of fasting are far reaching and exceptionally effective. This suggests to me that for people who are suddenly presented with an ailment, doing a two-week water-only fast, followed by a whole-food plant-based diet, is as good as it gets in terms of recovery and ongoing wellness.

As I mentioned, I was not familiar with the health benefits of fasting at the time I encountered my problem. I'd like to think that I was professionally prepared for these successes, but I simply did not realize they would be so profound. Without a doubt, this clinical intervention warrants far more attention in the healthcare system, and Dr. Goldhamer merits recognition as the dean of this discipline.

I highly recommend this book on fasting with no hesitation whatsoever. In a word, it is superb.

T. Colin Campbell, PhD

JACOB GOULD SCHURMAN PROFESSOR EMERITUS OF NUTRITIONAL BIOCHEMISTRY, CORNELL UNIVERSITY
COAUTHOR OF *THE CHINA STUDY*

[2] Goldhamer A, Lisle DL, Parpia B, Anderson SV, Campbell TC. Medically supervised water-only fasting in the treatment of hypertension. *J Manip Physiolo Therap* 2001.

PREFACE

Fasting is a very popular topic these days. How popular? According to Google Trends, interest in fasting tripled between 2013 and 2023, and there are more than 500 million websites covering topics including fasting for religious reasons, fasting to lose weight, fasting diets, and juice fasting. The historical, scientific, and clinical accuracy of these articles varies wildly. A few are written by experienced clinicians and scientists, but many more are written by people who have recently heard about fasting and are simply excited about it. Despite the differences in quality between these articles, they share a common thread: most of the writers have little or no clinical experience with the kind of prolonged water-only fasting that leads to significant reversal of disease. As a result, these articles are of little help to people seeking information about recovering from serious health problems. The purpose of this book is to provide the missing information that you and your doctor need to reap the maximum benefits of fasting.

Can Fasting Save Your *Life?* is born from the cumulative clinical experience gained by TrueNorth Health Center clinicians who, overseen by Alan Goldhamer, DC, since 1984 have successfully supervised more than 25,000 patients through prolonged water-only fasts lasting up to 40 days. This unparalleled clinical experience informs, and is informed by, the clinical research conducted by Toshia Myers, PhD, director of the TrueNorth Health Foundation since 2015. This book describes select classic and cutting-edge fasting research, concepts, and data, including a discussion of the clinical trials and case reports published by the TrueNorth Health Foundation in peer-reviewed journals. Most importantly, it examines how dietary pleasure can trap people into overeating, leading to excess fat gain, in particular visceral fat. This, in turn, promotes fatty liver, systemic inflammation, and insulin resistance, which set the stage for heart disease, diabetes, autoimmune disorders, and several forms of cancer. Moreover, this book describes the remarkable capacity of fasting to reduce fat, including visceral fat, and to lower biomarkers of fatty liver, systemic inflammation, and insulin resistance. In these ways, fasting may thereby allow our cells, tissues, and organs to recover from conditions that are conventionally considered unresolvable. A detailed overview of the science of fasting presents a clear path to understand how this natural approach can be used to restore and maintain health.

But please don't take our word for it. Read the book, apply the principles, and learn for yourself the remarkable benefits of fasting.

Toshia Myers, PhD

DIRECTOR, TRUENORTH HEALTH FOUNDATION

Alan Goldhamer, DC

DIRECTOR, TRUENORTH HEALTH CENTER

ACKNOWLEDGMENTS

This book was truly a team effort, especially on behalf of the TrueNorth Health Foundation employees Sahmla Gabriel, MUDr; Evelyn Zeiler, PhD; and Natasha Thompson, ND, whose contributions made this project possible, and for whom we are extremely grateful. We are also incredibly grateful for critical recommendations and revisions by David Goldman, MS, RD, CSCS, CPT; Jennifer Marano, DC; James Michael Lennon; Justin Wise, ND; Cheryl Steets; Larry Gitlin; and Patricia Kolbe, MS.

Introduction

Americans are in an alarmingly poor state of health, and we are not alone. Poor health is a massive problem worldwide. The combination of excessive calories, inadequate physical activity, and the increasing use of legal and illegal drugs has coalesced into one of the greatest noncommunicable disease crises in history. In the United States alone, more than half of adults—more than 150 million people—suffer from chronic diseases, and millions more have excess body weight. The vast majority of people also take prescription drugs in order to manage disease symptoms. The fact that the number of chronically ill, drug-dependent people is at an all-time high, despite record-breaking amounts of money spent on healthcare, provides strong evidence that pharmaceutical-based medicine is not the solution to our current health problems. If anything, harms caused by the over prescription and misuse of pharmaceutical drugs have contributed to the worsening health of millions of Americans. The likelihood of living with lifelong debility is a bleak reality for far too many people.

Maybe you are already healthy and are reading this book for insight into how to stay that way. If so, congratulations! Prioritizing your health now will help you retain your health into old age. More likely, though, you or your loved ones are among the majority of people who are chronically sick, and you are reading this book for insight into how to restore health. If so, congratulations to you too! As long as you are still alive, you can prioritize basic health practices that are foundational to a healthy life. But be forewarned: if you plan to fast, get "cured," and go right back to the habits that made you sick in the first place, you will likely be very disappointed. If you are willing to prioritize the behaviors that can enable you to live your precious life without ubiquitous aches and pains, joint replacements, heart surgeries, and pill popping, then this book will be a treasure trove of knowledge and inspiration that can support you on your journey.

Can Fasting Save Your *Life?* is more than just a catchy book title. It is a question asked in earnest. "Can fasting save *your* life?" Whether you are healthy or sick, when you undertake a prolonged water-only fast, it affects your entire physiology and benefits accrue beyond your control. Nonetheless, the answer still depends on you because only *you* can decide to fast, only *you* can prioritize time to fast, only *you* can make the diet and lifestyle changes necessary to sustain the benefits of fasting, and only *you* can resolutely continue making decisions that support your health throughout your life.

Fasting is not a one-off therapy or treatment, and it is certainly not a "cure" for anything. Periodic fasting, like exercising regularly, consistently getting sufficient sleep, or adopting a health-promoting diet, is a simple (albeit challenging) practice that is well within your reach. Yes, it's unusual, but so is exercising regularly, consistently getting sufficient sleep, and adopting a health-promoting diet. While less common than these other behaviors, water-only fasting just so happens to virtually reverse the chronic diseases many of us are suffering from, and it does so more effectively than many of the more common pharmaceutical and lifestyle interventions used today.

For convenience of language, throughout the book we refer to the "therapeutic" benefits of prolonged water-only fasting, but it must be understood that it is the human body, not the act of temporarily abstaining from food, that accomplishes the healing and recovery.

Health through Healthful Living

It is well documented that the best way to build and maintain good health is by living healthfully: eating a whole-food diet, staying hydrated, avoiding drug and alcohol abuse, getting sufficient physical activity and sleep, getting sufficient sun exposure and time in nature, reducing chronic stress, and sustaining meaningful connections with family and friends. Ideally, we would spend our entire lives prioritizing these healthful practices, thereby avoiding chronic disease altogether. However, the reality is that most of us spend our lives caught in a dietary pleasure trap and eventually develop one or more chronic diseases before we even reach old age. Fortunately, adhering to a healthy diet and lifestyle can help stop, and frequently reverse, the disease process. Even with this awareness, it can be difficult to break habits and make necessary changes. Thankfully, prolonged water-only fasting can help us accomplish this intimidating feat and jump-start the transition back to health.

Prolonged water-only fasting requires that we stop eating and drinking everything except water for an extended period, usually 2 to 40 days. It may sound preposterous to say that simply not eating for a period of time could help save our lives. But after four decades of supervising the fasts of more than 25,000 patients, we know that prolonged water-only fasting followed by controlled refeeding consistently produces beneficial outcomes in overall health and well-being. People of all ages, from all over the world, come to the TrueNorth Health Center with complaints of being obese or having chronic pain and fatigue, high blood pressure, and many other ailments. In the span of two to six weeks, they consistently see outstanding improvements in their clinical parameters of health. For most of our patients, total body weight typically drops by about 10%, blood pressure drops to within normal range without medications, and chronic pain naturally subsides. It is worth mentioning that in all of those fasts throughout the years, there has never been a single death associated with prolonged water-only fasting while under medical supervision at TrueNorth Health Center.

Throughout this book, we will share some extraordinary stories of patients who resolved health issues ranging from chronic post-traumatic headache to follicular lymphoma and eye degeneration. Some patients have reported feeling better than they have in decades. Others have had tumors go into remission. These cases represent just a few of the remarkable stories that illuminate the tremendous potential of prolonged water-only fasting followed by an exclusively whole-plant-food diet to help patients recover from myriad conditions. And although fasting is not a panacea, the overwhelming majority of our patients experience overall improvements in their health.

Besides sharing our patients' successes, we will also present a concise overview and history of fasting, introduce the physiology that determines why the foods we eat are so important, explain how a dysfunctional metabolism underlies various cardiovascular and metabolic diseases, review some of the latest human fasting physiology data indicating that fasting is safe, share promising evidence from the latest clinical research—especially with regard to reversing obesity and hypertension—and describe the future of prolonged water-only fasting in clinical research and practice, including the ways in which fasting benefits already healthy people. Finally, we will conclude with a detailed water-only fasting protocol that you can share with your physician (though training in the art and science of fasting supervision is highly recommended before a physician oversees such interventions) and provide information on some of the most supportive health practices available.

It has taken us almost a lifetime to accumulate this information, and we are excited to share it with you so that you can better understand how fasting, along with dietary and lifestyle changes, truly can save your life.

CHAPTER 1

A Primer on Therapeutic Fasting

Fasting is the partial or total cessation of caloric intake. And it is widely acknowledged that throughout human history people across cultures have independently practiced different types of fasting for a variety of reasons. It is intriguing that, even though eating and drinking are some of our greatest pleasures and just the thought of going without food can evoke our innate fear of starvation, fasting has endured for millennia as a means to exercise discipline, deepen spirituality, make a political statement, and improve health.[1] To this day, humans remain fascinated by the health-promoting effects of fasting. But why, exactly, has fasting persisted in each of these contexts? Why is fasting so meaningful to us when food is essential to our survival?

This book aims to address a key dimension of this meaningfulness by illustrating the therapeutic potential of water-only fasting. We make a case, based on scientific evidence and clinical experience, that therapeutic fasting continues to be used to maintain and restore health because it really does maintain and restore health. But the physical effects are just one aspect of fasting. Fasting, in particular prolonged water-only fasting, endures in part because it facilitates an enhanced sensory experience. The profundity of this experience undoubtedly comes from our heightened ability to perceive the dynamic physical, psychological, and metaphysical experiences that spontaneously and simultaneously occur during the fasting process. This natural intelligence is both universal and highly individualistic. It is also difficult, if not impossible, to quantify, and it is equally hard to capture with words. Undeniably, the best way to appreciate it is to undertake a prolonged water-only fast yourself (if clinically indicated, of course).

Fasting Is Not Starvation

Although you can find plenty of old and new scientific literature with the terms *fasting* and *starvation* used interchangeably, they are not synonymous. The terms indicate distinctly different physiological processes: Fasting is characterized by a decline in glucose metabolism and an increase in fat metabolism. Starvation, on the other hand, is characterized by a decline in fat metabolism and an increase in the synthesis of new glucose from recycled cellular material, including protein. Having enough energy is so critical that under conditions of extreme caloric restriction, this "recycled material" may be acquired by the breakdown of essential tissue, such as heart muscle. This typically occurs in the context of wasting syndrome, characterized by depletion of fat and other nutrient reserves, in late-stage terminal diseases or other circumstances of prolonged, extreme caloric restriction. In other words, starvation is a state of nutritional deficiency in which the body uses essential tissue for energy, and it is always harmful. Starvation could potentially occur in an improperly supervised or unsupervised fast, but prolonged water-only fasting—the focus of this book—is intended to be a temporary state of no caloric intake, in which the body uses excess fat for energy, and it is often therapeutic.

At this moment in history, we are collectively interested in the therapeutic aspect of fasting, and many people—ourselves included—are actively trying to harness the intelligence that is so readily activated by fasting to improve human health. Although the term *fasting* encompasses an entire continuum of methods, ranging from overnight fasting that naturally occurs during sleep to willfully abstaining from all food and liquid for consecutive weeks, there are only two categories of therapeutic fasting: intermittent fasting (IF) and prolonged fasting (PF). Within both categories there are several different types and several ways of practicing each type.[2] One thing that all types of fasting should have in common is reducing glucose utilization and increasing fat metabolism (i.e., ketosis) to one degree or another. In this chapter, we will briefly review the types of therapeutic fasting—other than prolonged water-only fasting—that are regularly used today.

Intermittent Fasting

Intermittent fasting (IF) is currently the most widely researched, publicized, and practiced method of fasting. The main types of IF include

TABLE 1.1. **Therapeutic fasting**

FASTING TYPE/ CATEGORY	FASTING DURATION	FASTING FREQUENCY	FASTING DIET
Time-restricted eating/IF	12 to 20 hours	Daily	Nothing (e.g., Ramadan fasting) Water, or water and acaloric beverages
Alternate-day fasting/IF	Up to 36 hours	Every other day	Water, or up to 500 kcal per fast
Twice-weekly fasting/IF	2 consecutive days or two 24- to 36-hour periods	Weekly	Up to 500 kcal per fast day
Fasting-mimicking diet/PF	5 consecutive days	Monthly for 3 months	1,100 kcal on the first day and 700 to 800 kcal on days 2 through 5
Minimally supplemented fasting/PF	5 to 21 days	As needed	75 to 250 kcal-per-day liquid diet
Water-only fasting/PF	Up to 40 days	As needed	Water Vegetable broth as needed

time-restricted eating (TRE), alternate-day fasting (ADF), and twice-weekly fasting (TWF). These methods have defined fasting periods lasting from 12 to 48 hours that are typically repeated on an ongoing daily or weekly basis. Although there have been hundreds of IF clinical research studies, which generally last 8 to 12 weeks, differences in study design, a lack of studies in populations with specific diseases, a lack of follow-up data, and difficulty with adherence make it challenging to translate study results into clinical treatment protocols. And it is unknown whether sex, age, or health status affect outcomes. For example, it was recently noted that there are differences between men and women during Ramadan fasting, a subtype of TRE, with diabetic women experiencing higher rates of low blood sugar than diabetic men.[3,4] Given the heightened interest in IF, more research is likely forthcoming.

Time-Restricted Eating

Time-restricted eating (TRE) involves eating within a specified period and abstaining from caloric intake (i.e., fasting) for the rest of the day.

Ramadan Fasting

During the month of Ramadan, Muslims undertake a daily fast during which no foods or liquids should be consumed from sunrise to sunset. Ramadan fasting, a type of religious fasting, was probably the first IF method consistently used by humans. There have been numerous clinical trials investigating the health effects of what is now referred to as Ramadan diurnal intermittent fasting (RDIF). Although recent reviews of RDIF research suggest that there are modest improvements in body weight and other biomarkers of cardiovascular and metabolic health, this research is difficult to interpret because outcomes are dependent on variables such as geographical location and the food and liquids consumed during the eating period.[50]

TRE is practiced daily with the rationale that nearly all organisms, including humans, operate within the context of a circadian rhythm that is approximately 24 hours long. Throughout this 24-hour cycle, human cells—through complex signaling pathways—anticipate changes in light, temperature, and nutrient intake in order to initiate metabolic and hormonal changes based on the predictability of these events. That means there are optimal times within the 24-hour cycle to sleep, eat, and exercise.[5]

The TRE window for food consumption generally ranges from 6 to 10 hours each day, and the fasting window comprises the remaining 14 to 18 hours. A typical schedule is 8 hours of eating and 16 hours of fasting, but some studies report an eating window as short as 4 hours or as long as 12 hours. The eating window may also be restricted to certain times of the day (e.g., early, middle, late). To date, there does not appear to be a consensus on an optimal length or time of day for eating since most studies have allowed for self-selected eating windows with various time periods. Studies comparing restricted eating to unrestricted eating during the eating window are also lacking.

Regardless of whether the fasting period occurs early or late, individuals following TRE regimens typically lose 1% to 4% of their initial body weight over an 8- to 12-week period. A growing body of research suggests that, despite minimal weight loss, TRE (particularly early day TRE) may offer other benefits, such as improvements in insulin resistance, systemic inflammation, and other markers of metabolic health.[6-10] Many of the purported benefits of TRE have been identified in animal models and need to be verified in humans.

Caloric Restriction

Caloric restriction is a method of eating in which daily caloric intake is consistently lower than the amount needed to maintain weight, but not so much as to cause malnutrition. Although caloric restriction is inherent to prolonged water-only fasting, it is not synonymous with fasting because there are some intermittent fasting (IF) methods (e.g., time-restricted eating) that do not necessarily result in caloric restriction. Caloric restriction was popularized after reports that it increased life span by as much as 300% and improved biomarkers of inflammation, metabolism, and stress response in animal models.[51,52] Yet there are valid criticisms. For example, it can be difficult to meet nutrient requirements in humans and outcomes are overblown because the control animals were permitted unrestricted access to food; that is, the experiments were comparing calorically restricted populations to overfed, rather than normally fed, populations. Nonetheless, these findings ignited interest that led to the expansive body of IF research available today.

Alternate-Day Fasting

As the name suggests, alternate-day fasting (ADF) alternates between one "fast" day and one "feast" day. The fasting day is either 100% caloric restriction, which consists of drinking only water and other noncaloric beverages (e.g., black coffee and tea), or significant caloric restriction (i.e., modified ADF), which consists of consuming approximately 500 or fewer calories per day, or only 25% of daily caloric intake. The feast day allows for unrestricted eating. The rationale is that alternate-day fasting, which requires caloric restriction only every other day, is more feasible than daily caloric restriction.

ADF was first studied in mice as an alternative to chronic caloric restriction. There have recently been several larger meta-analyses of the numerous individual studies reporting on the effects of ADF. A meta-analysis of seven randomized controlled trials lasting from 4 to 48 weeks with populations that included normal, overweight, and obese participants found that ADF caused modest improvements in body weight, body mass index, total cholesterol, low-density lipoprotein, triglycerides, and resting blood pressure when compared with a control population with no dietary restrictions. There were no differences in blood glucose or biomarkers of insulin resistance between these populations.[11] Another meta-analysis found similar results: overweight adults who followed an ADF regimen for at least 6 months reported an average weight loss of 5.8 pounds.[12] However, an umbrella analysis of systematic reviews and meta-analyses of ADF research revealed that nearly all of the findings were of low or moderate quality,[13] with only one study producing high-quality evidence indicating that 1 to 2 months of modified ADF resulted in an average reduction of 1.2 points in body mass index.[11]

Twice-Weekly Fasting

Twice-weekly fasting (TWF), otherwise known as the 5:2 diet, includes five days of unrestricted eating and two days of consuming 25% of total energy requirements, approximately 500 calories per day. The "fasting" days, with significant caloric restriction, can be either consecutive or nonconsecutive. Although there are fewer research studies investigating the effects of TWF, the human health benefits appear to be similar to those of other IF methods. A recent comprehensive synthesis of systematic reviews and meta-analyses found that after 3 months, TWF resulted in statistically significant weight loss of 3.7 pounds that was sustained for the next 6 to 12 months. There was also limited evidence that 3 to 6 months of TWF reduced insulin resistance in overweight and obese women when compared with caloric restriction alone.[13]

Prolonged Fasting

Prolonged fasting (PF) consists of partial or total caloric restriction for up to 40 days. The main types of PF are minimally supplemented fasting (i.e., Buchinger fasting) and water-only fasting, which are both well-established therapeutic interventions that clinical research is only beginning to validate. The fasting-mimicking diet (FMD), the third type of PF, was developed by gerontologist and biologist Valter Longo, PhD, and is now established as a medical intervention. Research into FMD methods is rapidly expanding, but there are currently very few randomized controlled trials exploring their effects on human health. Despite this dearth of research, there may be advantages to undergoing PF rather than caloric restriction or IF methods. For example, the average prolonged fast may be more feasible because it does not require months of caloric restriction or ongoing, repeated, short fasting intervals. Furthermore, PF typically lasts 5 to 21 days, which provides individuals with an opportunity to break habits and improve their adherence to healthy behaviors after the fast. For example, at least 5 days of PF may increase fruit and vegetable consumption.[14]

Fasting-Mimicking Diet

Fasting-mimicking diets (FMDs) are designed to mimic PF methods by increasing ketone levels without completely eliminating caloric intake. FMDs typically provide 1,100 calories on the first day and 700 to 800 calories on days 2 to 5 with a macronutrient breakdown of 9% to 10% protein, 50% to 60% fat, and 30% to 40% carbohydrates.[15] Proponents of FMDs argue that they provide the benefits of PF without the risk, but there are currently no studies comparing the relative safety or effectiveness of FMDs with other types of PF. There have been numerous studies on FMDs in rodent animal models. Mice fed FMDs are reported to experience health benefits, such as regeneration of tissue and organs, reduced measures of inflammation, increased insulin sensitivity, improved cardiac health and cognitive performance, decreased incidence of cancer, and extended health span.[16]

There have also been numerous clinical trials, and there are currently more randomized FMD controlled trials (completed or underway) than any other PF method. One of the first clinical trials in overweight but otherwise healthy humans found that three consecutive cycles of FMDs with unrestricted eating in the non-fasting period were able to reduce body weight, body mass index, blood pressure, and abdominal circumference, all while preserving lean mass, compared with a control group that continued normal eating behavior. The average weight lost was 5.7 pounds.[17] A recent study of the effects of cyclic FMDs in conjunction with traditional cancer therapies in 100 patients with various types of cancer reported a reduction in body mass index, blood glucose, insulin, and circulating insulin-like growth factor 1 in these patients as well as improved anticancer immunity in breast cancer patients.[18]

The ProLon Fasting Mimicking Diet, developed by Dr. Longo, is the first commercially available FMD and is gaining recognition in mainstream medicine.[19] Meals and beverages include dried soups, olives, and proprietary bars, drinks, and dietary supplements without a strict schedule for consumption. Periods between these five-day diets allow for unrestricted eating. It is recommended that the ProLon diet be used for no more than three consecutive months. If health goals are met, it is suggested that patients consider repeating the cycle every three to six months. Patients who do not meet their health goals should consider completing one or two additional consecutive cycles and then repeat the cycle every three to six months. Research exploring the long-term outcomes of this extended intervention is lacking.

Minimally Supplemented Fasting

Minimally supplemented fasting is a type of PF during which patients consume 75 to 250 calories of freshly prepared juice and vegetable soup per day for up to 21 days, and sometimes longer. The most popular and researched type of minimally supplemented fasting is the Buchinger fasting method, which was developed by Otto Buchinger and described in his book *The Healfast*, published in 1935. In Germany and Spain, there are Buchinger Wilhelmi clinics, which offer a comprehensive, multidimensional program with dietary, physical activity, communal, mindfulness, and psychological components.[20]

In the past several years, Françoise Wilhelmi de Toledo, MD, who is married to Dr. Buchinger's grandson Raimund Wilhelmi, and her group have published numerous clinical and physiology studies on the effects of this type of PF in humans. These studies, some with sample sizes of more than 1,000 people, have contributed greatly to our knowledge of PF in normal-weight, overweight, and obese people, as well as in healthy and unhealthy people.[21-32]

The data indicate that minimally supplemented fasting is well tolerated and has a low incidence of adverse side effects, which mainly include mild headache, lower backache, and a moderate amount of sleep disturbances within the first days of fasting.[32] Furthermore, research indicates that protein utilization moderately increases during the early stages of fasting but decreases after day five as levels of ketones rise.[23] George F. Cahill Jr., MD, and colleagues found similar results regarding protein catabolism in research conducted during prolonged water-only fasting decades ago.[23,33] Reductions in body weight, body mass index, waist circumference, blood pressure, blood glucose, fatty liver index, heavy metals, and blood lipids were also reported with an average of 10 days of minimally supplemented fasting.[24,26,30] For example, 20 days of this fasting regimen resulted in an average weight loss of 19 pounds.[34] Overall, minimally supplemented fasting appears to improve markers of cardiovascular and metabolic health similar to other fasting methods.

Water-Only Fasting

Water-only fasting, the focus of this book, is a type of PF in which only water is consumed for up to 40 days, typically while under medical supervision. The fasting period is necessarily followed by a controlled refeeding period of at least half of the fast's length. Prolonged water-only fasting is often referred to as zero-calorie fasting or total fasting and inaccurately as periodic fasting, which is a misnomer since PF does not necessarily need to be repeated.[35] It is also sometimes mistakenly called "starvation," which is an entirely different physiological process.[36] Since 1984, the TrueNorth Health Center (TNHC) has implemented a prolonged water-only fasting protocol based on the protocol developed by the late 19th- and early 20th-century hygienic physicians. This protocol is also the method used in research conducted at the TrueNorth Health Foundation (TNHF). There are other prolonged water-only fasting protocols that appear in the scientific literature, including beego fasting, which originated in China approximately 2,500 years ago.[37,38]

Given the long history of prolonged water-only fasting, it is unsurprising that there are more than 600 published case reports and observational water-only fasting studies in humans. Many of these studies indicate that this type of PF is also beneficial to health.[37-47] Furthermore, a recent randomized controlled trial found that six days of water-only fasting improved glucose tolerance and insulin secretion better than two days of fasting, suggesting that PF may have advantages over shorter fasts.[48] Despite this long-standing interest by the medical and scientific communities, there is still a lack of randomized controlled trials comparing prolonged water-only fasting with other fasting methods or standard medical interventions for the treatment of any disease. Future research may explain the relationship between prolonged water-only fasting, self-healing, and any long-term health benefits.

Conclusion

Fasting is a potential solution to the current problem of chronic overconsumption and the resultant high rates of cardiovascular and metabolic diseases. It appears that all types of IF and PF—including TRE, ADF, TWF, FMD, minimally supplemented fasting, and water-only fasting—result in beneficial physiological changes. However, there are still many unanswered questions, especially about the magnitude of these changes and whether they produce long-term health benefits. It is also unknown whether age, sex, and health status impact outcomes and how the various fasting methods compare with one another and with the standard treatments of care used in mainstream medicine. We may learn that the best outcomes result from approaches that use a combination of these methods, depending on the needs of specific patients. In the following chapters, we will detail the physiological rationale for why the ancient practice of water-only fasting is a potential solution to prevalent metabolic health problems. In chapter 2, we will give a brief historical review of therapeutic water-only fasting.

CASE SUMMARY

Seborrheic keratosis lesion resolves from woman's face after prolonged water-only fasting followed by a salt-, oil-, and sugar-free diet.

Seborrheic keratosis (SK) is a benign skin tumor with unknown etiology that affects more than 90% of adults over age 65. Although benign, SK lesions often continue to grow unless they are removed for medical or cosmetic reasons. Current FDA-approved treatments for SK are cryotherapy, electrocautery, and 40% hydrogen peroxide. Noninvasive treatment options do not exist. We published a case in *Alternative and Complementary Therapies* demonstrating that an SK lesion that had been growing on a patient's face for 10 years resolved with water-only fasting and an exclusively whole-food plant-based diet free of added salt, oil, and sugar (SOS-free diet).[49]

A 68-year-old woman came to TNHC with the intention of treating obesity, hypertension, and diabetes. She also had a 0.4 x 0.4-inch SK lesion on the right side of her face that had appeared 10 years earlier and had continued to grow and change in shape and color. Despite these changes, she was denied reimbursement for medical treatment because the lesion was benign.

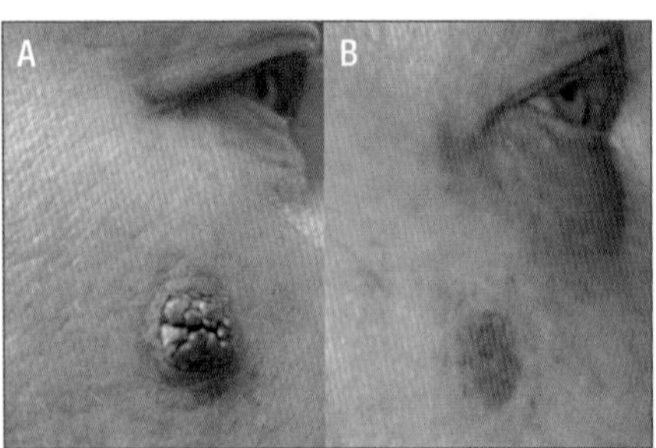

FIGURE 1.1. Seborrheic keratosis on right cheek (A) before treatment and (B) after treatment.

Upon arrival, the patient was examined and approved for a water-only fast. She began her treatment by eating an SOS-free diet at TNHC for 7 days and then completed 11 days of water-only fasting followed by another 10 days of an SOS-free diet. Surprisingly, within the first 7 days on the diet, the patient reported that the SK lesion had started "crumbling off" while she washed her face and that this continued throughout her stay. Unsurprisingly, at the end of treatment, she had lost 10% of her total body weight, her unmedicated blood pressure was 111/75 mmHg, and her fasting blood glucose dropped 66 points to within normal range. When the patient returned to TNHC about eight months later to continue treatment for cardiometabolic disease, she reported that two weeks after her last visit, the SK lesion had completely "fallen off" (see figure 1.1).

This report demonstrates how water-only fasting and an SOS-free diet results in whole-body changes, such as reduced measures of systemic inflammation, that can lead to unexpected outcomes and may hold potential as a low-risk treatment for SK.

CHAPTER 2

The Origins of Water-Only Fasting in the United States

When the term *fasting* is used in this book, it refers to prolonged water-only fasting: or a period of time when someone with enough nutrient reserves voluntarily stops eating and drinking everything except for pure water for 2 to 40 days. Many people understandably think that 40 days is an absurdly long time to go without food. Yet humans are so well adapted to fasting that some people can consume only water for two to three months without entering starvation.[1] Survival during caloric deprivation hinges on an ability to metabolize different fuel sources (i.e., sugar, fat, and protein) depending on our nutrient status, which is variable and dynamic.

This metabolic flexibility needed to adapt to fasting evolved in single-cell organisms billions of years ago.[2] Human metabolic flexibility involves a fairly well defined series of metabolic adaptations that begin early in the fasting process (see chapter 4), but it is the ability to burn fat stores for energy that is the key to our survival. From this perspective, it is easy to see how an ability to store fat that can be used for energy when food is scarce may have conferred a strong survival advantage.[3] Especially considering that humans lived as hunter-gatherers with inconsistent access to food and most likely experienced prolonged periods without caloric intake for essentially all of our 200,000-year history.

For at least 2,500 years, the word *fasting* has been used to describe restricted caloric intake under vastly different circumstances, and ancient historical texts indicate that humans have a long and varied cultural relationship with fasting and have used it for political, spiritual, religious, and therapeutic reasons.[4] For example, fasting in various forms has a long history in Western and Eastern religions such as Christianity, Islam, and Buddhism, and there are types of religious fasting that involve total abstinence from food and drink during a specific time of the week or year. Because the topic is vast, and religious and political fasting have been extensively reviewed elsewhere, in this chapter, we will focus on the history of the medically supervised prolonged water-only fasting method, including how it was developed at the TrueNorth Health Center (TNHC) and how it is being researched at the TrueNorth Health Foundation (TNHF).

Fasting for Health

The use of fasting to improve physical health is not new. Evidence dating back more than 2,000 years reveals that ancient Greek scholars, including Plato and Hippocrates, practiced and promoted therapeutic fasting.[5] China's history of therapeutic fasting goes back more than 2,000 years and was described in *The Yellow Emperor's Classic of Medicine*, the earliest encyclopedia of traditional Chinese medicine written during the Western Han dynasty (202 BCE to 9 CE).[6]

Throughout the past 200 years, therapeutic fasting has gone in and out of fashion with both allopathic and alternative health practitioners in Europe and the United States. In recent decades, therapeutic fasting has resurfaced as a possible antidote to contemporary health issues that largely result from the overconsumption of processed foods. We will proceed with a brief historical account of the development of prolonged water-only fasting currently used in clinical practice at TNHC and the focus of the research conducted by TNHF.

In the 19th century, a group of physicians began exploring the possibility of a scientific alternative to the random and sometimes crude attempts to cure disease being practiced by their contemporaries. They recognized that common medical practices, including bloodletting and snake oil consumption, were unable to help those in need, as empirical data would later confirm. Through their clinical experience and careful study of anatomy, physiology, and pathology, these physicians came to formulate the basic principles of what became known as hygiene, the science of health. The principles of hygiene directly address the inherent physiological requirements to sustain health: proper nutrition, fresh water, physical activity, rest, sunshine, fresh air, and emotional composure. Furthermore, hygiene was built on the basic assumption that, when each of these needs are met, humans have an innate ability for self-regulation and healing.

The pioneer of the hygiene movement, which largely brought therapeutic fasting to the United States, was the Yale-educated medical doctor Isaac Jennings (1788 to 1874).[7] The story goes that he grew increasingly disillusioned with regular medicine and, after 20 years of practice, abandoned it for a hygienic practice. Jennings did not believe that all disease symptoms were inherently problematic and should therefore be suppressed. Rather, he saw many of them as remedial processes through which the body regained its health, processes he believed should be respected and supported. Therefore, he encouraged self-healing through hygienic dietary and lifestyle practices, combined with the judicious use of water-only fasting.

Jennings was a major influence on Sylvester Graham (1794 to 1851), a Presbyterian minister and temperance lecturer who inspired others to bring health education to the public in the early 19th century. In contrast to the prevailing medical recommendations of the times, Graham advocated a diet of fruits, vegetables, and whole grains; exposure to fresh air, pure water, and sunlight; exercise and nonrestrictive clothing; and the habit of bathing.[8] He also championed women's rights and the abolition of slavery. In time, more and more physicians centered their practices on hygienic principles. Prominent among them were William Andrus Alcott, MD (1798 to 1859); Thomas Low Nichols, MD (1815 to 1901); Susanna Way Dodds, MD (1830 to 1911); and Russell T. Trall, MD (1812 to 1877). By the early 20th century, the fundamental principles of hygiene were diluted in a variety of nontraditional therapeutic schools and alternative treatment approaches.

Although the teaching and practice of hygiene continued at various clinics for many years, it fell out of practice, replaced largely by more conventional medicinal approaches. This led Herbert Shelton (1895 to 1985) to research and organize the fundamental principles of hygiene into a cohesive body of knowledge. He called this approach "natural hygiene" to distinguish it from the general practices of sanitation and personal hygiene that were linked to an array of questionable therapies and schools of his day. Shelton was one of the most prolific writers and teachers of hygienic living and is credited with reviving the hygiene movement. Besides establishing a fasting institution and health school, he wrote many books as well as a monthly hygiene magazine.[9] In addition to his own work, Shelton collected and preserved hundreds of books written by 19th-century hygienists. These books now constitute the Herbert Shelton Collection at the H.J. Lutcher Stark Center for Physical Culture and Sports (Stark Center) at the University of Texas at Austin. In 1948, Shelton, along with a few like-minded physicians, founded the National Health Association (then known as the American Natural Hygiene Society), a lay organization dedicated to preserving the tenets of hygiene and the benefits, research, and practice of medically supervised water-only fasting.

The Beginning of Fasting Research

Over the past several years, there has been an increased interest in the clinical effects of prolonged water-only fasting, and many original research studies have been published. Although it appears that we have entered a new era, research into the clinical effects of water-only fasting in humans actually has a long and curious history that, like the study of hygiene, began in the late 19th century. At the time, it was common for men known as "hunger artists" to undertake prolonged water-only fasts in public for both amusement and profit. These stunts garnered a lot of interest, but the artists were frequently suspected of being fraudulent, and they received considerable scrutiny from the public as well as medical and scientific professionals. Remarkably, fasting publicity stunts still occur. In 2003, David Blaine conducted a 44-day water-only fast and remains a notable example of how inappropriate eating after fasting may result in potentially fatal refeeding syndrome[10] (see chapter 8).

As interest in hunger artists grew in the 19th century, so did the interest in the use of experimental research to gather objective data on human physiology. Medical doctors and scientists seized the opportunity to study physiology in these professional fasters. In 1888, Luigi Luciani (1840 to 1919) conducted one of the first public experimental investigations of hunger artist Giovanni Succi, who performed at least thirty 30-day public fasts.[11] This collaboration was purportedly mutually beneficial as it helped Luciani substantiate his unified theory of physiology and disproved claims that Succi was a fraud. Eventually the overall interest in hunger artists waned, as did the practice of publicly conducting experimental research on fasting men. But this was just the start of clinical research into the effects of water-only fasting, and more would soon follow.

In 1915, Francis Gano Benedict (1870 to 1957) published the first controlled observational investigation of a man who fasted for 31 days in the Nutrition Laboratory in Boston.[12,13] Many similar studies were published throughout the early 20th century. Then interest waned until 1959, when Walter L. Bloom (1915 to 2007) published the article "Fasting as an Introduction to the Treatment of Obesity."[14] This, in turn, prompted research into the clinical effects of water-only fasting in obese subjects that continued into the late 1970s. Clinical research declined following this period, in part due to reports of serious complications, including death, in some fasting subjects. These deaths were almost certainly due to harmful fasting practices, including arbitrarily implementing fasts lasting 60 days or longer and intravenously administering nutrients, such as electrolytes and protein, in order to artificially prolong fasts.[15] Additionally, physicians and researchers did not always screen subjects for contraindications, nor did they terminate fasts upon complication or properly refeed subjects, all of which are necessary procedures for the safe implementation of prolonged water-only fasts.

In the 1960s, a group of researchers led by diabetes expert George F. Cahill Jr. (1927 to 2012) began investigating human metabolism during fasting. They conducted human research examining various physiological changes that occur during fasting.[16] This research continued into the late 1990s. During this time, researchers discovered that during prolonged water-only fasting, ketones supply approximately 66% of the brain's energy requirements.[17] These contributions are a tremendous source of our current knowledge on glucose, fatty acid, and amino acid metabolism and organ function during the fasting process. Recently, there have been a handful of physiology studies reexamining metabolism during fasting that support and expand on the original research.[18-20] By the late 1970s, it became clear that fasting research was valuable, but guidelines and standards for interventional protocols were needed to ensure the safety of study participants.

In 1978, the International Association of Hygienic Physicians (IAHP) was formed to establish training requirements and professional standards for water-only fasting interventions and, more broadly, to promote hygienic lifestyle practices. To this day, IAHP provides training and examination to certify clinicians in prolonged water-only fasting supervision. This training has proven invaluable for the safe and effective operation of the few prolonged water-only fasting centers that exist around the world (see the list at fasting.org). Of these, the TNHC is the largest residential facility, providing 24-hour medical supervision of fasts lasting 2 to 40 days.[21] TNHC was founded in 1984 and is located in Santa Rosa, California. Since its inception, clinicians at the center have supervised the fasts of more than 25,000 patients, and the center currently accommodates more than 1,200 patients each year. In addition to treating patients, TNHC is the only center that trains clinicians to become IAHP-certified in prolonged water-only fasting supervision.

TNHF, founded in 2011, is a clinical research institution developed primarily to expand evidence-based knowledge of how prolonged

Timeline of Prolonged Water-Only Fasting in Medicine and Research

Early to mid-1800s: Isaac Jennings was credited as the first US physician to use therapeutic fasting and hygienic lifestyle practices. Sylvester Graham, a Presbyterian minister and temperance lecturer, popularized fasting and hygienic lifestyle practices.

Late 1800s: "Hunger artists" undertook prolonged water-only fasts in public for amusement and profit.

1888: Luigi Luciani, a prominent Italian physiologist, conducted some of the first public experimental investigations of hunger artist Giovanni Succi's prolonged water-only fasts.

1915: Francis Gano Benedict, a chemist, physiologist, and nutritionist, published the first controlled observational investigation of a man who underwent a water-only fast for 31 days at Boston's Nutrition Laboratory.

Mid-1900s: Herbert Shelton, a chiropractic and naturopathic doctor, was credited for reviving the hygiene movement, including the use of water-only fasting.

1948: The National Health Association was founded.

1959–1970s: In the article "Fasting as an Introduction to the Treatment of Obesity," Walter L. Bloom, a medical doctor and scientist, catalyzed inquiry into the clinical effects of water-only fasting in obese subjects.

1960s to late 1990s: George F. Cahill Jr., a medical doctor and biochemist, and others investigated metabolism and organ function during the fasting process, contributing tremendously to our current knowledge.

1978: The International Association of Hygienic Physicians was founded to establish training requirements and professional standards for the conduct of water-only fasting and to promote hygienic lifestyle practices.

1984: The TrueNorth Health Center was established.

2003: David Blaine, a performance artist, undertook a 44-day public water-only fast for entertainment and developed refeeding syndrome.

2011: The TrueNorth Health Foundation was established.

2018: TrueNorth Health Foundation published the first comprehensive safety analysis of prolonged water-only fasting.

water-only fasting impacts human health. TNHF's ever-growing list of completed clinical trials and peer-reviewed publications have contributed to the current understanding of fasting physiology and its potential to reverse some of the most common chronic diseases. TNHF also trains clinical research scientists, funds clinician training, and publicly shares findings and resources (see fasting.org). Importantly, TNHF is one of the few institutions that investigates the refeeding period and beyond, which is essential in distinguishing between acute physiological adaptations and sustained health outcomes. The results of this and other research will be presented throughout this book.

Conclusion

Humans have a time-honored and multifaceted relationship with fasting. We appear to have fasted since time immemorial for reasons as varied as food scarcity, religion, spirituality, entertainment, and medical therapy. This is made possible by our ability to metabolize fat for energy, and as such, even prolonged water-only fasting can usually be accomplished without adverse effects. Fortunately, despite historical periods when fasting was unpopular, our knowledge of safe fasting practices has persisted, enabling qualified medical professionals to support most people through a prolonged water-only fast lasting up to 40 days. The following chapters will highlight our current understanding of the physiological and clinical benefits of fasting, review the current research, and discuss unanswered questions about how research may improve the practice of therapeutic fasting. We will begin with a detailed look at evidence showing that prolonged water-only fasting is safe when conducted properly.

CASE SUMMARY

Uncomplicated subacute appendicitis managed with prolonged water-only fasting in an adult male.

Our studies show that fasting may not only reverse obesity and other chronic diseases caused by poor diet and lifestyle—the focus of this book—but also improve acute conditions. We published the following case report in the *Journal of Alternative and Complementary Medicine* of a patient diagnosed with appendicitis who, instead of having the recommended surgery, opted to undertake a prolonged water-only fast followed by an exclusively whole-plant-food diet free of added salt, oil, and sugar (SOS-free diet).[22] Appendicitis is a sudden inflammation of the appendix that rapidly worsens and is potentially fatal, but this very rare case was feasible because the patient never developed a fever and his pain did not worsen, more consistent with a subacute clinical picture.

A 46-year-old man arrived at the TNHC reporting that he'd had pain in the lower right quadrant of the abdomen for three days. He denied having had any pain or bleeding with urination, nausea, vomiting, or diarrhea. He did not have a fever but did have a tender, nonprotruding mass in the lower right quadrant. The patient was advised to obtain a surgical consult, during which the surgeon concluded that there was no hernia present and advised the patient to use nonsteroidal anti-inflammatory medication and to return for further consultation if his pain worsened or if a bulge developed.

One month later, the patient returned to TNHC, reporting increased pain during his activities of daily living. He still denied nausea, vomiting, constipation, and diarrhea and did not have a fever. His physical exam revealed slight tenderness on the lower right quadrant of the abdomen but no palpable mass. Ultrasound showed an enlarged, noncompressible appendix with increased blood flow along the periphery, all signs of appendicitis. The patient was advised to have his appendix surgically removed (which has been the standard treatment for appendicitis since the late 1800s). He refused and opted to try prolonged water-only fasting before considering surgery.

Upon approval, he fasted for seven days, followed by four days of supervised refeeding with a controlled SOS-free diet, and he was monitored twice daily throughout the intervention so that the supervising physician was regularly updated of the patient's health status.

The patient remained afebrile with a normal white blood cell count throughout treatment and reported reduced abdominal pain during the refeeding period. The patient continued to follow the recommended diet and had follow-up visits regularly for three months, during which he reported that he was without abdominal pain and had returned to his daily activities, including physical exercise. At his two-year follow-up visit, he reported continuing the diet and lifestyle recommendations and remaining completely free of abdominal pain. This report describes a single case of uncomplicated subacute appendicitis that was successfully managed with fasting and diet; it is not a blanket recommendation but rather a glimpse into the unexpected ways that prolonged water-only fasting may benefit health.

CHAPTER 3

Hard Evidence That Fasting Is Safe

Humans can safely undertake prolonged fasts because of our ability to metabolize both sugar (i.e., glucose) and fat (i.e., fatty acids) to meet our energy needs, and an average-size person is estimated to have sufficient nutrient reserves to water-only fast for up to two, maybe up to three, months before entering starvation.[1,2] Indeed, there are numerous documented examples of people safely fasting for up to 40 days and even a published case report of an artificially prolonged, supervised fast lasting 382 days, during which a 27-year-old man weighing 456 pounds successfully reduced his body weight by more than half.[3] Yet, even after millennia of therapeutic use and more than a century of published research, prolonged water-only fasting has not gained widespread acceptance by medical and scientific professionals and is still frequently criticized as an unfeasible and dangerous intervention.[4-6] This skepticism contrasts with the popularity of intermittent fasting, which has become widely accepted in recent decades. In many ways, it is understandable why people choose intermittent fasting over a more intensive intervention: prolonged water-only fasting requires one to six weeks of residential medical supervision, and the mere thought of spending many days without eating and drinking anything but water can provoke a primal fear of starvation, which will certainly occur if one stops caloric intake for long enough. Although we acknowledge that unsupervised fasting can be dangerous, the focus of this chapter is to present another perspective.

Consider that the prolonged water-only fasting protocol detailed in this book has been safely used in clinical practice for at least a century and at the TrueNorth Health Center (TNHC) for more than 40 years. As such, contraindications to fasting are already well established.

Current protocols monitor for and attend to any side effects, effectively helping patients avoid potentially serious problems. Furthermore, clinical research is beginning to validate what has been witnessed in the clinic for decades: many people are *willing* and *able* to fast and experience only minimal transient side effects, which pale in comparison to the overall benefits they incur. For example, a recent study assessing the safety of fasting in people with high blood pressure found that more than 95% of participants reported preferring fasting to using medication (see chapter 6). Fasting not only lowered their blood pressure (as happens with medications[7]) but also improved their overall health. What's more, residential treatment, which some people view as inconvenient, can actually prove to be tremendously helpful in establishing new behaviors that support long-term success, such as breaking unwanted habits, learning new lifestyle skills, allowing a repose from stress, and building social connections with like-minded people.

Safety is another reason for the common yet unsubstantiated belief that all forms of extended fasting are inherently dangerous. And while it's true that medical supervision has not always been a guarantee of safety, in reality there have been only 19 published reports of serious adverse events during prolonged water-only fasting in either clinical practice or clinical research. Consider what happened in the 1950s to 1970s, when an extreme form of medically supervised prolonged water-only fasting was used for weight loss, mostly in cases of severe obesity.[8] During this time, supervising clinicians engaged in some unintentionally harmful fasting practices. Some clinician researchers commonly reported high rates of weight loss, but a few also reported serious adverse effects, including death.[9-11] For example, in one case, an obese man with a preexisting heart condition (now considered a contraindication to fasting) went into cardiac arrest and died during his third week of fasting.[12] The serious adverse events and deaths reported during this time most certainly could have been prevented with more appropriate fasting supervision.

Fortunately, today there is an accepted way to characterize the safety of fasting (or any medical intervention for that matter). This established method involves regularly monitoring, measuring, and recording acute signs, symptoms, and biomarkers of health. Reported symptoms, heart rate, blood pressure, and blood glucose are recorded in accordance with the Common Terminology Criteria for Adverse Events (CTCAE), which was established by the National Cancer Institute for reporting adverse events during cancer drug trials.[13]

What Is an Adverse Event?

An adverse event is an unfavorable symptom or laboratory finding during a medical treatment (e.g., pharmaceutical drugs) or procedure (e.g., surgery). Adverse event reporting during clinical trials can help assess the safety of an intervention. The Common Terminology Criteria for Adverse Events established by the National Cancer Institute has standardized terminology for adverse event reporting in clinical research.[43] Adverse event terms are grouped by system organ classes (e.g., nervous system) and presented with a 0 to 5 grading scale, indicating a range from no adverse events to death. A serious adverse event is an event that results in hospitalization or extension of hospitalization, a substantial reduction in ability to conduct activities of daily living, or death.

Physiological Evidence That Fasting Is Safe

To determine for yourself whether fasting is safe, it is necessary to have a basic understanding of how fasting affects essential physiological functions. As mentioned earlier, there is an established protocol for assessing acute health status throughout the fasting process (also see chapter 8). This protocol includes, but is not limited to, daily interviews and physical examinations and at least weekly urine and blood testing. Systematically recorded clinical information can then be used to characterize adverse events.

In this chapter, we will discuss commonly assessed acute biomarkers of health. Since the initial changes that occur during early phase fasting (i.e., intermittent fasting research) have been described elsewhere,[4,6,14-18] we will give a brief overview of select changes that occur specifically during prolonged water-only fasts lasting at least five days when steady-state fasting begins. When possible, data collected during and after refeeding will also be described. These time points are critical for determining whether existing changes revert or additional changes occur after fasting has concluded.

Vital Signs

Vital signs are objective measures of essential physiological functions, such as body temperature, respiration rate, heart rate, and blood pressure. Vital signs, along with information about symptoms (e.g., fatigue) and behaviors (e.g., physical activity), are checked twice daily during medically supervised fasts to help clinicians assess overall health. Available data indicate that, during water-only fasts lasting 10 or more days, there is essentially no change in body temperature or the percentage of peripheral oxygen saturation.[1,2,7] Heart rate increases slightly (by approximately 0.5 beats/minute) but stays within normal range and decreases again after refeeding.[7,19,20] There are also significant reductions in resting blood pressure, but systolic/diastolic blood pressure very rarely drops to below 90/60 mmHg, which is actually a safe blood pressure reading and may also confer health benefits.[7,19,21] In steady-state fasting that typically occurs by day 7, vital signs tend to remain stable.

Complete Blood Count

A complete blood count (CBC) is routinely measured at annual physicals and during fasting to explore common physiological changes. Recent research has confirmed that, during water-only fasts lasting at least 10 days, some components of the CBC fluctuate, but all median values stay within normal range (see appendix 5).[7,19,20] Notably, white blood cells (and especially neutrophils, which are markers of immune function) significantly decrease during fasting. These white blood cells remain below pre-fast levels through the end of refeeding and return to pre-fast levels within six weeks.[7,19,22]

Electrolytes and Other Blood Chemistry

The comprehensive metabolic panel (CMP) includes 14 different blood tests that assess electrolytes, glucose, liver and kidney function, and other parameters of overall health. Recent studies assessing electrolyte levels during prolonged water-only fasting report that several blood electrolytes (including magnesium, potassium, phosphate, sodium, bicarbonate, chloride, and calcium) fluctuate, but the changes are usually mild (e.g., sodium and potassium may drop to 130 mEq/L or 3.0 mEq/L, respectively) and revert to pre-fast levels with refeeding.[7,19,22,23] (A complete list of blood count and chemicals and symptoms that indicate potentially serious deviations are described in appendix 5.) Most of these changes are not problematic unless accompanied by physical symptoms. Notably, markers of liver and kidney function may temporarily increase within normal range during fasting and revert to pre-fast levels or better within six weeks.[7,19]

Electrolytes are minerals such as sodium, potassium, and magnesium that maintain homeostasis by regulating fluid levels, nutrient cycling, waste removal, and other processes. A common concern about prolonged water-only fasting surrounds the potential for electrolyte imbalance. These concerns are not completely unfounded, given that hyponatremia (low sodium in the blood) is a potentially serious problem that is easily corrected if swiftly identified.[21] Recent studies assessing electrolyte levels during prolonged water-only fasting report that several blood electrolytes (including magnesium, potassium, phosphate, sodium, bicarbonate, chloride, and calcium) fluctuate but typically remain within normal range and revert to pre-fast levels with refeeding.[7,19,23] Transient changes in hydration and electrolytes are common throughout the day even while eating, depending on a number of factors, but fluctuations are usually not a cause for concern in the absence of physical symptoms.

During fasting, there are many other changes in blood chemistry, including the characteristic decrease in glucose that typically stays above the lower limit of normal and eventually returns to pre-fast levels with refeeding. During a 10-day fast, there is no change in water-soluble vitamins, but as may be expected from increased fat metabolism, the concentration of fat-soluble vitamins (A, D_3, and E) in the blood increase. The concentration of fat-soluble vitamins in the blood return to pre-fast levels upon refeeding.[19]

Refeeding syndrome is a critical imbalance in cellular concentrations of electrolytes, including potassium, sodium, or thiamine (vitamin B_1), that can occur within the first 3 days of refeeding, especially in cases of malnutrition that occurs after prolonged periods of extreme caloric restriction brought on by chronic disease or other involuntary circumstances.[24,25] Although refeeding syndrome is also possible after prolonged water-only fasting, the syndrome is essentially unheard of during controlled refeeding after medically supervised fasts. Furthermore, a recent study found that 3 days after a 10-day water-only fast, electrolytes (e.g., sodium and phosphate) and vitamins (e.g., thiamine) were within normal range.[19] There are a few case reports of people who undertook unsupervised prolonged fasts of 40 days or longer and developed Wernicke encephalopathy, which is a degenerative neurological disorder caused by thiamine deficiency during refeeding due to uncontrolled food reintroduction.[26-30] There have been no instances of refeeding syndrome during controlled refeeding at TNHC.[21]

Uric Acid

Although it is well known that uric acid increases beyond normal levels during fasting, the increase is not typically associated with physical symptoms and reverts with refeeding. Older fasting studies, and even a recently published one, report preemptively "treating" high uric acid with the popular anti-gout drug allopurinol.[31] The rationale for artificially lowering uric acid is to avoid a hypothetical episode of gout. Yet despite the fact that nearly everyone experiences an increase in uric acid, there are essentially no new cases of gout during fasting; thus, allopurinol is not indicated or used in current protocols. The increase in uric acid during prolonged water-only fasting could even be a beneficial adaptive mechanism, because uric acid has the ability to increase sodium retention and maintain blood pressure during periods of caloric deprivation.[32] Uric acid also promotes tissue remodeling by increasing immune cell response and reducing free radicals.[33]

Blood Lipids

Blood lipids, including total cholesterol, high-density lipoprotein, low-density lipoprotein, very low-density lipoprotein (VLDL), and triglycerides fluctuate in response to prolonged fasting, depending on an individual's starting weight. Recent studies of fasts lasting at least 10 days suggest that total cholesterol does not change in overweight or obese people with high-normal cholesterol and actually increases in normal-weight people with normal cholesterol. The reasons for these differences are unknown, but by the end of the controlled refeeding period, total cholesterol levels decrease to slightly below starting levels in both normal-weight and obese populations, which is a beneficial outcome. VLDL and triglycerides also increase during fasting and controlled refeeding but revert to starting levels within six weeks.[7,34,35] These peripheral increases likely have to do with increased production and transport of triglycerides bound to VLDL during fasting and a lag during the metabolic switch from ketosis to glycolysis.[35]

Body Weight and Composition

Weight loss during fasting is well characterized; the rate of weight loss is approximately 2 pounds per day, ranging from about 4 pounds per day for up to approximately one week, after which it reduces and plateaus at less than a pound per day as fasting progresses over 30 days.[1,7] Within two weeks of fasting, overweight and obese people lose an average of 10% total body weight, and normal-weight people lose an average of 7%. Total weight increases slightly (< 2%) during initial food reintroduction with the replenishment of glycogen and accompanying fluid stores. This rate of weight loss is comparable to other accepted weight-loss strategies that are considered safe, such as bariatric surgery, which results in an average of 6% weight loss within two weeks of surgery, and very low-calorie diets, which result in rates of loss of approximately 1.6 pounds per day.[36,37]

Dual-energy x-ray absorptiometry (DXA) technology (a type of low-radiation X-ray) provides a convenient and accurate measure of total body composition. A few studies have used DXA scans to assess changes in fat and lean mass after prolonged water-only fasting. Although these studies report varying fast lengths and population characteristics, the general trend is a 10% reduction in lean mass (including fluid loss) and 10% to 20% decrease in total fat in approximately 6 to 11 days of fasting. Remarkably, fat mass, including estimated visceral fat, continues to decline throughout the immediate food reintroduction period.[7,19] Depending on fast length and body type, total visceral fat loss has been reported at 12% to 50%.[7,38] Importantly, total lean mass was reported to increase with food reintroduction and reverts to near pre-fast levels within six weeks, even in the absence of resistance exercise training programs such as weight lifting or calisthenics. These data indicate that fasting does not result in sustained losses in lean mass.

Clinical Evidence That Fasting Is Safe

Remarkably, despite centuries of contention and decades of clinical data collection, the safety of medically supervised prolonged water-only fasting was not assessed in a peer-reviewed publication until 2018, when John S. Finnell and colleagues published a large retrospective safety study that directly investigated the adverse events experienced during prolonged water-only fasting at TNHC.[21] This landmark study described the adverse events that occurred over five years and 768 patient visits. The study subjects completed water-only fasts lasting from 2 to 40 days and a controlled refeeding period of half the fast length. Adverse events were categorized according to the CTCAE described earlier.[13]

The study found that most patients experienced at least one adverse event during the fasting period (*N* = 686/758; 91%). The highest-grade adverse events were overwhelmingly mild to moderate and already known to commonly occur during fasting (e.g., nausea, back pain, headache, and presyncope). In the visits in which the highest-grade adverse events were severe (*N* = 184/758; 24%), more than 40% were high blood pressure events in patients who had a preexisting hypertension diagnosis, suggesting that the rate of treatment-emergent severe adverse events is even less than reported. There were two serious adverse events (one case of dehydration and one case of low sodium) that occurred in men in their early seventies. Both required intravenous treatment with saline solution, and both resolved without further complication. Increased fast duration was not associated with increased adverse-event severity, as underscored by the fact that one of the serious adverse events occurred on the third day of fasting. Importantly, there were zero deaths in this study, and there has never been a death associated with more than 25,000 prolonged water-only fasts undertaken at TNHC.

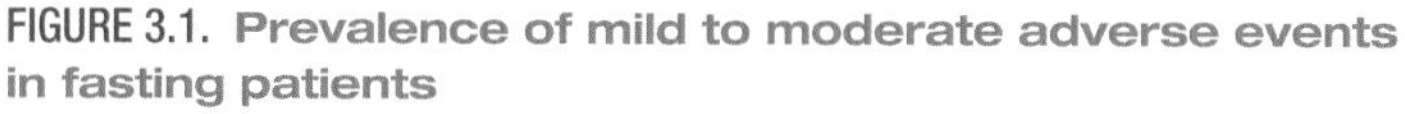
FIGURE 3.1. **Prevalence of mild to moderate adverse events in fasting patients**

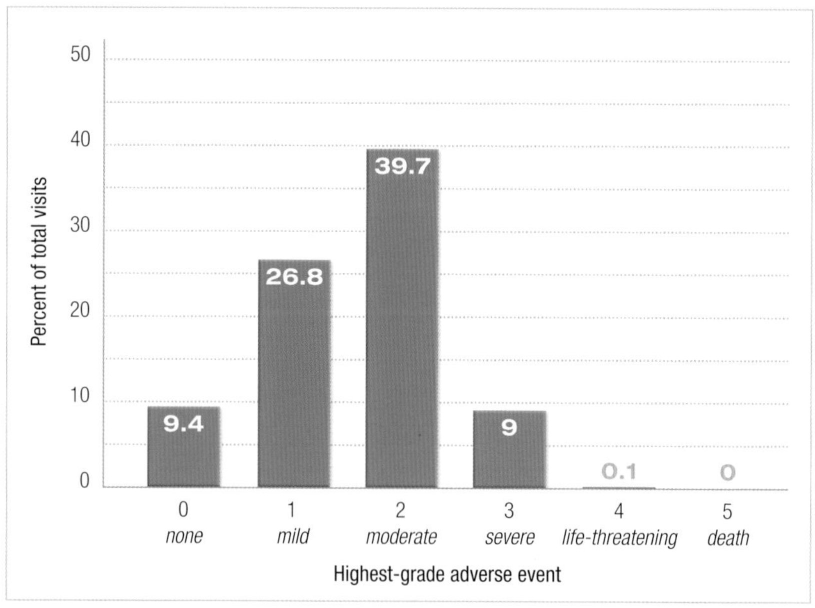

Note: Severity and occurrence of adverse events (listed according to the Common Terminology Criteria for Adverse Events) during prolonged water-only fasting lasting 2 to 41 days with an average of 7 days.[13]

The TrueNorth Health Foundation (TNHF) recently completed a prospective safety study, specifically in people with hypertension who fasted for an average of 11 days.[7] Adverse events found in this much smaller study were similar to those found in the larger retrospective analysis—namely, that 76% (*N* = 22/29) of participants experienced mild to moderate adverse events, such as transient fatigue, nausea, and insomnia. There were no serious adverse events or unresolved complications due to fasting. This study also included an analysis of numerous blood variables, such as electrolytes and markers of liver function, and the results are in agreement with data from existing publications.[19,20,22,23]

TNHF has published prospective data on more than 100 research volunteers who fasted an average of 14 days.[7,34,35,39] In all these fasts, the vast majority of events were mild and already known to commonly occur during prolonged water-only fasting, and there were no serious adverse events. There also have been more than 100 publications in the 21st century documenting more than 2,000 fasts conducted at in-patient facilities around the world, and there have been only 12 reports of transient serious adverse events.[21,26-28,30,40,41] The most serious reports involved people who fasted on their own and developed Wernicke encephalopathy or electrolyte imbalance during unsupervised refeeding.[26,28]

The data from these studies overwhelmingly support that medically supervised prolonged water-only fasting can be safely practiced in a residential setting. However, reports of serious adverse events underscore the importance of fasting under medical supervision, especially for those who have medical conditions or need to wean off medications. Our recommendation is that people undertake a prolonged water-only fast only under the medical supervision of an expertly trained fasting supervisor using a validated protocol.[21] Anyone who wishes to take or supervise a water-only fast should confirm that there are no contraindications and be aware of the potential symptoms, especially serious adverse events such as electrolyte imbalance and dehydration. Fortunately, qualified clinicians trained in fasting supervision have access to an already well-defined list of contraindications and side effects (see chapter 8). It is important that researchers and clinicians continue closely monitoring and accurately reporting adverse events associated with water-only fasting. This is especially critical with regard to specific populations, such as people with kidney disease.

Conclusion

Fasting is a well-tolerated, integrative process that is adaptive, progressive, and dynamic. It is remarkable that a treatment with so much therapeutic potential has so few serious or sustained side effects. It is also notable that most adverse events are mild complaints such as fatigue, insomnia, and nausea. This is especially significant since the adverse event data come from TNHC patients, a population that typically begins fasting with multiple chronic conditions and complaints. Compound that with the discomfort of suddenly (or even gradually) stopping the consumption of food and harmful substances (such as alcohol and caffeinated drinks), which are common coping mechanisms, and it can be a difficult mental and physical transition. Yet decades of clinical practice have consistently demonstrated that people can cope with discomfort, and the side effects eventually subside. Although it is imperative that clinicians and researchers continue to monitor and publish on adverse events that can occur during prolonged water-only fasting, for most people, the benefits appear to far outweigh the marginal risks.

CASE SUMMARY

Woman experiences long-term relief from chronic post-traumatic headache after two 40-day water-only fasts and an exclusively whole-plant-food and salt-, oil-, and sugar-free diet.

We published a case in *Alternative and Complementary Therapies* demonstrating that a woman who completed two medically supervised prolonged water-only fasts with a six-month intervening period, eating an exclusively whole-plant-food diet free of added salt, oil, and sugar (SOS-free diet), gradually eliminated a case of unrelenting bilateral chronic post-traumatic headache (CPTHA).[42] This is a remarkable example of not only what is possible with repeated periods of prolonged fasting but also the art and science of fasting supervision.

A 58-year-old woman arrived at TNHC with an incessant, moderate-to-severe bilateral headache that began 16 years earlier, after she was hit in the head with a metal bar. She was diagnosed with CPTHA, which occurs in 20% to 95% of people who have suffered a traumatic brain injury (TBI), potentially due to long-term neurogenic inflammation and lack of effective intervention. She was also diagnosed with chronic pain and thoracic outlet syndrome and had been prescribed a variety of pharmaceuticals, including gabapentin, topiramate, pregabalin, desvenlafaxine, and acetaminophen with codeine, without achieving any significant pain relief. She became interested in water-only fasting after she learned of the potential to reduce her brain inflammation.

The patient was approved to undertake a medically supervised prolonged water-only fast that lasted 41 days without serious adverse events. On day 37, she reported that the intensity and duration of head pain had decreased (see table 3.1). During the 20-day refeeding period, she reported that the daily headaches were of much lower intensity, and she experienced pain-free periods. She also reduced from the obese to overweight category. The pain relief was substantial enough that she decided to continue eating the SOS-free diet after she returned home.

Six months later, the patient returned to TNHC and completed another 40-day water-only fast followed by 20 days of refeeding. On arrival, she was of normal weight and experiencing moderate headaches lasting no longer than 15 minutes daily. Toward the end of treatment, she no longer experienced daily headaches, and the headaches she did have were mild and lasted less than 10 minutes. The patient continued with an SOS-free diet and, at her three-month follow-up visit, had maintained normal weight and reported that the headaches were mild and infrequent. Remarkably, at a five-year follow-up visit, she reported

TABLE 3.1. **Immediate and long-term effects of fasting and diet on CPTHA, BMI, and BP**

	FAST #1		FAST #2		FOLLOW-UP	
(Ref. range)	Day 0	Day 37	Day 0	Day 37	3 months	5 years
HA intensity (0-10)	6-8/10	3/10	6/10	1/10	1/10	1/10
HA duration (0 min–constant)	Constant	< 1 h	≥ 15 min	< 10 min	< 10 min	< 10 min
HA frequency (never–daily)	Daily	Daily	Daily	Infrequent	Infrequent	Infrequent
BMI (18.5–24.9 kg/m^2)	33.1	26.9	23.7	18.8	20.2	22.1
SBP (90–120 mmHg)	118	106	98	78	92	106
DBP (60–80 mmHg)	78	64	68	65	58	67

Note: BMI, body mass index; BP, blood pressure; DBP, diastolic blood pressure; HA, headache; kg, kilogram; m, meter; min, minutes; mmHg, millimeters of mercury; SBP, systolic blood pressure.

that the headaches remained mild and infrequent. She had also maintained normal weight (see table 3.1).

This case sets a tremendous precedent for further inquiry into sequential, prolonged water-only fasting as a potential treatment for TBI-induced CPTHA. It is remarkable for other reasons too. It demonstrates that a well-selected, medically supervised patient can complete two 40-day fasting periods within one year without serious complications. It also suggests that sufficiently motivated patients can tolerate prolonged fasting periods and, perhaps most extraordinarily, commit to the long-term dietary adherence necessary to reverse obesity and maintain normal weight.

CHAPTER 4

Fasting Reverses Metabolic Dysfunction

Human diets have almost always consisted of various combinations of carbohydrates (i.e., glucose), fats (i.e., fatty acids), and proteins (i.e., amino acids) as well as vitamins and minerals from whole foods found in nature that required a lot of energy to procure. Food availability has historically alternated between periods of abundance and periods of scarcity, and humans are metabolically adapted to thrive under both conditions.[1] Processed foods—which are cheap to produce and contain artificially high concentrations of carbohydrates, fats, and nonnutritive chemicals—were introduced about 100 years ago and today comprise more than half of all food consumed in the United States.[2] We are not metabolically adapted to this new environment, as underscored by rates of chronic diseases that are at an all-time high.

Diet is significant because our bodies need correct amounts of macro- and micronutrients to maintain metabolic homeostasis, or balance. This balance guarantees that each cell has the right amount of energy and the building blocks necessary to carry out essential processes, like protein synthesis. Ensuring that our cells function optimally by consuming natural whole foods and getting physical activity is important because cells form the tissues, which form the organs and organ systems that, together, make up the totality of our bodies. Although humans have an obligatory need for nutrients, we can survive for prolonged periods with nothing but water because of our ability to store relatively large amounts of fat and use it instead of glucose to meet most of our energy needs. This metabolic adaptation also contributes to the reversal of detrimental metabolic effects caused by overconsumption of highly processed foods. Although this explanation oversimplifies incredibly complex biological phenomena, it does help illustrate how the foods we eat (and don't eat) contribute to our overall health.

In this chapter, we will describe how our bodies metabolize food, how we adapt throughout the fasting process, and how our metabolisms malfunction with overconsumption. We will include clinical data that indicates how a single three-week fasting and refeeding intervention begins to reverse early stage metabolic dysfunction, providing encouragement for people diagnosed with metabolic syndrome or type 2 diabetes mellitus. We hope this knowledge inspires you to consider fasting as a way to begin rebalancing your metabolism, make better lifestyle choices, and ultimately improve and sustain your health.

Metabolism

The term *metabolism* collectively describes the catabolic and anabolic biochemical reactions that are essential to life. Catabolic reactions break down larger molecules into smaller ones, *creating* energy in the form of adenosine triphosphate (ATP) in the process. Conversely, *anabolic* refers to reactions that build larger molecules from smaller ones, *consuming* ATP energy in the process. In this way, catabolism provides the building blocks and energy needed to create complex molecules (such as nucleotides, peptides, lipids, and polysaccharides) that are used during anabolic processes, including DNA replication and the biosynthesis of hormones, enzymes, and neurotransmitters.[3]

Human cells, like the cells of all living organisms, require building blocks and energy to complete obligate physiological functions. Our primary source of these starting materials are the nutrients we absorb from our diet. Nutrient metabolism begins with digestion, which breaks down the carbohydrates, fats, and proteins into glucose, fatty acids, and amino acids that are taken up by cells for use in subsequent metabolic processes.

The liver is one of the most metabolically active organs in the body. When functioning optimally, it helps maintain nutrient homeostasis by metabolizing, storing, or releasing glucose, fatty acids, and amino acids. This is a highly complex process with many regulatory factors, including the concentration of available and stored nutrients, the relative concentrations of hormones (e.g., insulin, glucagon), and the metabolic activity of other organs and tissues (e.g., brain, skeletal muscle, adipose tissue). In metabolically healthy individuals, glucose, fatty acid, and amino acid metabolic homeostasis ensures that whole-body energy requirements are met.[4-6]

When nutrients (primarily glucose) are depleted, several metabolic adaptations occur in order to metabolize fat stores that supply the energy needed to keep our tissues and organs functioning and ensure our survival. George F. Cahill Jr. and colleagues described these metabolic processes in five distinct phases based on blood glucose and ketone concentrations as well as rates of glucose and fatty acid metabolism.[7] Contemporary researchers have started using large-scale data analysis to better understand these processes based on the relative expression of metabolic proteins. This research has begun to redefine these phases,[8,9] but results are too preliminary to be conclusive. A sixth phase that seems to occur during the transition back to "fed" metabolism is also being characterized.[10,11] (You can stay up to date on the latest research at fasting.org.) The following explanation of metabolic phases I to V is complex and covers a lot of biochemistry, which some people may find difficult to follow.[12] If you prefer to jump straight to reading about how fasting improves metabolic health, go to page 49.

Fed Metabolism

Metabolic Phase I

Phase I begins with digestion immediately following caloric ingestion, when carbohydrates, fats, and proteins are catabolized into sugars, free fatty acids and glycerol, and amino acids, respectively. Glucose and amino acids are absorbed directly into the bloodstream through the small intestine. Free fatty acids and glycerol form micelles that enter cells of the intestinal lining (enterocytes), where they are reconverted to triglycerides/triacylglycerols (TAGs) and packaged in chylomicrons. Chylomicrons are absorbed into the lymphatic system through the small intestine and then released into the bloodstream.[13]

Glucose

All tissues, except the liver and heart, readily utilize glucose as fuel. Glucose is transported into cells, where it is catabolized through glycolysis. Glycolysis is the first of three steps that occur in cellular respiration. During glycolysis, which occurs in the cytoplasm, glucose is converted into two pyruvate molecules, releasing ATP and nicotinamide adenine dinucleotide (NADH) in the process. During the second step, which occurs in the mitochondrial matrix, pyruvate is oxidized into acetyl-CoA, an additional molecule of NADH, and carbon dioxide (CO_2). The acetyl-CoA is then used in the Krebs (TCA/citric acid) cycle to produce ATP and more CO_2, NADH, and flavin adenine dinucleotide ($FADH_2$). Finally, oxidative phosphorylation, which occurs in the mitochondria and includes the electron transport chain and chemiosmosis, uses the molecules of NADH and $FADH_2$ from the previous reactions to make water and much more ATP.[14] In total, one glucose molecule generates 38 molecules of ATP.

Glucose is either used to meet immediate energy needs (as described earlier) or taken up by the liver and skeletal muscles and converted to glycogen. This process is called glycogenesis, and it enables carbohydrate storage until peripheral glucose supplies need to be replenished. Glycogen is also used to meet the muscles' energy needs during physical activity, at which point it can be converted back to glucose in a process called glycogenolysis. The liver and skeletal muscles of an average-size, metabolically healthy person store approximately 100 and 500 grams of glycogen, respectively.[15] The brain also stores a small amount of glycogen, which is logical given its glucose requirements. Under fed conditions, insulin is secreted from the pancreas and regulates glucose metabolism by promoting cellular glucose uptake, suppressing glycogenolysis and gluconeogenesis (the de novo synthesis of glucose) in the liver, and increasing glycogenesis in the liver and skeletal muscle.[16]

Fatty Acids

Dietary fats are broken down into fatty acids and glycerol molecules and used to meet immediate energy needs or stored as TAGs. Three fatty acids and one glycerol combine to form one TAG molecule. TAGs are the storage form of fat and take the form of lipid droplets in the cytoplasm of most cells, most notably in adipose tissue. TAGs are used to meet energy needs and are essential during ketogenic conditions, including the overnight fast. To produce energy, TAGs are catabolized back into free fatty acids and glycerol. In a process called fatty acid oxidation, free fatty acids are bound to coenzyme A (CoA) and converted to fatty acyl-CoA in the outer mitochondrial membrane. This molecule is then transported to the inner membrane, where it combines with carnitine to form acylcarnitine. Acylcarnitine, in turn, is transported into the mitochondrial matrix, where it converts back to fatty acyl-CoA. At this point, fatty acyl-CoA can be used to generate ATP through beta-oxidation, which ultimately produces a molecule of acyl-CoA that is two carbons shorter and reenters beta-oxidation, as well as a molecule of acetyl-CoA that enters the Krebs cycle to create ATP. This cycle continues until the fatty acid substrate is catabolized. In total, this process creates 129 molecules of ATP, which is more than three times the amount that is created with cellular respiration, and it is a key reason why humans are so well adapted to store fat. In addition to meeting cellular energy requirements, fatty acids are used for other critical processes such as cell membrane synthesis and hormone regulation.

When nutrients are abundant, insulin suppresses lipolysis and prevents adipose secretion of TAGs. Insulin also regulates fat metabolism in the liver by suppressing fatty acid oxidation, increasing de novo lipogenesis, and inhibiting VLDL-TAG secretion to replenish liver fat stores for later use. Another way that insulin regulates fatty acid metabolism is by promoting the expression of lipase, an enzyme that breaks down TAGs in the bloodstream into fatty acids so they can be absorbed by muscle cells for energy production.[17] Human adipose tissue is able to store large amounts of TAGs, as evidenced by the current obesity crisis.

FIGURE 4.1. **Macromolecule metabolism and storage**

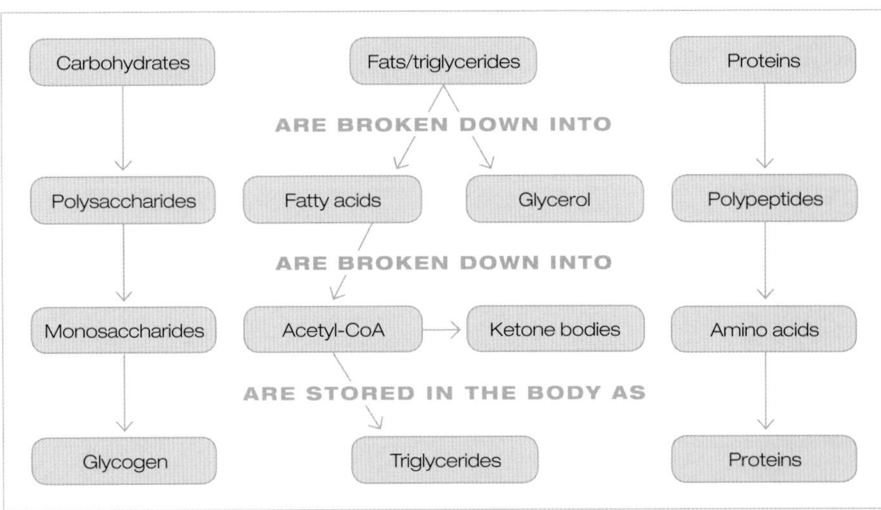

Note: Macromolecules are large molecules obtained from our diet that are essential for cell structure and function. In humans, carbohydrates are broken down into polysaccharides and then into monosaccharides for storage as glycogen for energy. Triglycerides, also known as fats, are broken down into glycerol and fatty acids, which are further broken down into acetyl-CoA, which can be converted into ketone bodies for use when glycogen is low or into triglycerides for long-term energy storage. Proteins are broken down into polypeptides and further into amino acids, which are utilized for various cellular functions and can be stored temporarily as proteins in the body.

Amino Acids

There are 20 amino acids, 9 of which are essential and must be obtained from our diet. The other 11 are also present in the diet but can be generated from glycolytic and Krebs cycle intermediates from glucose metabolism when necessary. The liver is the primary site of amino acid metabolism, but skeletal muscle also metabolizes amino acids and incorporates them as protein, which can be catabolized back into amino acids, if necessary. Amino acids are used in many processes, such as generating nitric oxide, neurotransmitters, and catecholamines or modifying genetic material. If free amino acids are not used, they are degraded into ammonium ions that enter the urea cycle and a carbon "skeleton." These are used to make Krebs cycle intermediates and generate ATP or in the de novo (i.e., from-scratch) synthesis of glucose (gluconeogenesis) or fatty acids (lipogenesis) for use or storage.[3]

Fasting Metabolism

Once we stop eating, blood glucose and insulin levels gradually drop, initiating the transition into fasting. When liver glycogen stores are depleted, blood glucose and insulin levels decline, and fatty acid and (eventually) ketone oxidation both increase to meet energy requirements. [7,12] These dynamic processes are regulated by numerous physiological adaptations that preserve essential organs and ensure that energy needs for the entire body are continuously met. For example, thyroid hormones respond quickly to fasting, including a decrease in T3 and TSH and an increase in free T4, but decrease to pre-fast levels upon refeeding.[18,19,20,21]

Metabolic Phase II

Phase II begins approximately 4 to 6 hours following final caloric intake and continues until liver glycogen is depleted. Decreased blood glucose levels stimulate pancreatic cells to secrete glucagon above basal levels. Glucagon, an insulin antagonist, stimulates glycogenolysis in the liver to produce glucose from stored glycogen. Liver glycogen reserves are depleted within approximately 24 hours of fasting during sedentary conditions or in the absence of exercise. During this early fasted phase, liver glycogenolysis provides about 75% of daily glucose requirements, and gluconeogenesis accounts for the remaining 25%. Glycogenolysis also converts muscle glycogen to glucose 6-phosphate.

However, muscle cells lack the enzyme glucose 6-phosphatase that is required to release glucose; therefore, muscle glycogen is not used to meet whole-body glucose requirements but rather remains in the muscle until it is required for forceful contractions. Leptin, which is considered an appetite suppressant, decreases by as much as 50% within the first 24 hours of fasting, and the reduction is sustained throughout the fasting period. The decrease in leptin is inversely correlated with a concomitant increase in cortisol.[22,23] This quick drop in leptin suggests that it is not responsible for fat loss; rather, it is the lack of leptin combined with increased cortisol that promotes the early fasting response to increase fat metabolism. Therefore, it appears that the increase in cortisol is an acute adaptive response and is not considered to be harmful in the same way that chronically high cortisol is. Adiponectin does not change during fasting or at least not in amounts detected in the peripheral blood.[24] Toward the end of this period, fatty acid oxidation is used to meet the majority of energy needs.[7,12,21]

Metabolic Phase III

Phase III generally lasts from 24 to 48 hours following final caloric intake. During this time, gluconeogenesis is the primary metabolic pathway supplying daily glucose requirements. Gluconeogenesis, which occurs primarily in the liver, produces glucose from glycerol, lactate, and amino acids. TAG hydrolysis forms fatty acids and glycerol in adipose tissue. Glycerol is converted to dihydroxyacetone phosphate, which is used to produce glucose in the liver, after which it is exported to other tissues. Amino acids are primarily used to make protein, but when glucose is low, glucogenic amino acids are used for gluconeogenesis. In skeletal muscle, ammonium is produced as a by-product of protein catabolism, but it cannot be converted to urea for removal through urine, as in the liver. Excess ammonium results in transamination of surplus pyruvate to ultimately form alanine. The glucose-alanine (or Cahill) cycle transports the glucogenic amino acid, alanine, from skeletal muscle to the liver to produce glucose that can then be used outside the liver. Although all amino acids, except lysine and leucine, are glucogenic, alanine and glutamine are the predominant amino acids used in gluconeogenesis in the liver and kidneys, respectively. Eventually, the kidney synthesizes more glucose through gluconeogenesis than the liver does. During this phase, fatty acids make more ATP than is made with glucose.[7,12,21]

Metabolic Phase IV

Phase IV begins approximately 48 hours and ends between five and seven days after final caloric intake. Throughout this phase, kidney gluconeogenesis becomes progressively more important in the maintenance of blood glucose levels. Reduced blood glucose and increased glucagon levels induce adipocytes to increase lipolysis of TAGs into free fatty acids and glycerol. Glycerol is converted to glucose through gluconeogenesis. Fatty acids bound to albumin are transported to the liver, muscle, and other tissues. Fatty acids in the liver are catabolized via beta-oxidation to form acyl-CoA and acetyl-CoA. When acetyl-CoA exceeds the capacity of the Krebs cycle due to reduced oxaloacetate availability, it is used to synthesize the ketones acetoacetic acid (AcAc), acetone, and beta-hydroxybutyric acid (βOHB) through ketogenesis.

The liver is unable to use ketones for fuel, which results in large quantities of ketones, primarily AcAc and βOHB, secreted into the bloodstream. Within the mitochondria of non-liver tissue, βOHB is further oxidized to AcAc, which enters the Krebs cycle, ultimately producing 22 molecules of ATP. Increased ketones are typically identified through urinalysis by day three of the fasted state. Except for red blood cells, the kidney medulla, and the liver, all other tissues—especially most of the brain—are able to utilize ketone for energy. After approximately four days of fasting, the brain begins utilizing ketone, primarily beta-hydroxybutyric, and ketosis provides the majority of the brain's energy requirements throughout the remainder of the fasting process.[25] This adaption is essential because the brain does not store large amounts of glycogen and requires approximately one-third of its fuel in the form of glucose.[7,12,21,26]

Metabolic Phase V

Phase V begins when rates of ketogenesis exceed gluconeogenesis. The urine concentration of ketones increases steadily from < 0.5 mmol/L while feeding, and it plateaus at > 16 mmol/L during this phase.[27,28] The rate of increase and the final concentration differ slightly based on individual characteristics (e.g., amount of lean versus fat mass). Notably, unlike the pathophysiology of type 1 diabetes, which also presents with high blood glucose levels, the high level of ketones observed during steady-state fasting is not associated with ketoacidosis.[29] The effects of increased exposure to ketones in humans from prolonged water-only fasting is still poorly characterized but may have health-promoting benefits.

Phase V is considered steady-state fasting, and the length of this phase depends on an individual's body mass index (BMI), fat and muscle mass, electrolyte stores, physical activity levels, and state of health. Studies on respiratory quotient and urinary nitrogen have demonstrated that adipose TAG stores contribute to more than half of whole-body energy requirements during this phase. Meeting energy requirements through fat metabolism decreases dependency on gluconeogenesis, thus sparing protein. The brain (40 g/day) and other tissues (40 g/day combined) still have an obligatory need for approximately 80 g/day of glucose, which is met through gluconeogenesis. Resting metabolic rate, which increases within the first three days of fasting, decreases below pre-fast levels by the ninth day and recovers upon refeeding.[19] If a person were to continue abstaining from food beyond their stored reserves, they would enter starvation. Starvation begins when rates of ketogenesis decrease and rates of gluconeogenesis increase, which indicates that essential protein is increasingly catabolized to meet energy requirements.[7,12,21] Current fasting protocols ensure that fasting concludes long before this point (see chapter 8).

Metabolic Phase VI (Refeeding)

Upon food reintroduction, blood ketone concentrations quickly revert to non-fasting levels, while blood glucose and insulin levels increase beyond pre-fasting levels.[30] Preliminary evidence suggests that, within six weeks of refeeding, insulin sensitivity increases slightly beyond baseline, reflecting favorable metabolic health.[10] Under normal conditions, temporary elevation of blood glucose and insulin concentrations may indicate reduced insulin sensitivity, but when this occurs in the context of the fasting process, it reflects a temporary adaptation that may facilitate the transition back to glucose metabolism. The mechanism by which this occurs appears to be entirely different from the pathophysiology of insulin resistance observed in the progression of type 2 diabetes.[11] Metabolic studies in humans during refeeding after prolonged water-only fasting are lacking, but the TrueNorth Health Foundation recognizes their value and investigations are forthcoming. Fortunately, the metabolic adaptations that occur during fasting begin to reverse the metabolic dysfunction caused by excessive sugar and fat consumption, which we will describe in the next section.[10,30]

What Is Insulin Resistance?

Insulin is a hormone produced by beta cells in the pancreas. Under normal fed conditions, insulin signaling promotes the uptake of blood glucose and free fatty acids into cells. Insulin-sensitive cells respond appropriately to insulin signaling and maintain metabolic homeostasis. A recent shift in perspective is that the interaction of insulin, glucose, and free fatty acids is collaborative rather than antagonistic, with fatty acids acting as a buffer to maintain glucose homeostasis.[37] In overfed conditions, impaired glucose and fatty acid metabolism leads to insulin-resistant cells that can no longer respond appropriately to glucose and free fatty acids. Since insulin is the primary hormone regulating glucose uptake into cells, when glucose levels exceed demand or glycogen storage capacity is reached, this leads to too much insulin production, or hyperinsulinemia.[48]

One hypothesis is that the cells become insulin resistant, or "unresponsive" to insulin, in order to counteract the high concentrations of insulin that drive more and more glucose and fatty acids into cells.[49] It may also be that insulin resistance contributes to hyperinsulinemia by necessitating increasing amounts of insulin to maintain blood glucose homeostasis.[49] Furthermore, when cells become unresponsive to insulin, lipolysis and de novo lipogenesis increase, eventually exceeding fat storage capacity and increasing adipose dysfunction as well. Excess blood lipids cause the liver and skeletal muscles to accumulate large amounts of ectopic fat, leading to lipotoxicity that exacerbates insulin resistance and inflammation through poorly defined mechanisms.[33,50] In this way, localized insulin resistance and inflammation lead to nonalcoholic fatty liver disease (NAFLD), systemic inflammation, hypertension, metabolic syndrome, type 2 diabetes, microvascular and macrovascular diseases, and other chronic conditions.[51]

Early insulin resistance is difficult to diagnose. It is typically identified based on clinical presentation of metabolic syndrome or insulin resistance syndrome once it is already established. Early assessment of insulin sensitivity could offer clues about overall metabolic health and help prevent disease as early as 10 years before its development. Currently, there is no standardized method of assessing early development of metabolic disease. However, validated indices, such as the homeostatic model assessment of insulin resistance (HOMA-IR), can be used as noninvasive screening tools in clinical practice to help promote early preventative interventions.[52]

Homeostatic Model Assessment of Insulin Resistance (HOMA-IR)

HOMA-IR uses fasting levels of glucose and insulin in the blood to predict both insulin resistance (IR) and beta-cell function.

A HOMA-IR value of 1 is assumed to be physiologically normal insulin sensitivity. Research is ongoing, but a value above 2.5 is generally accepted as characterizing an insulin-resistant state.[52]

Overfed Metabolism

Highly processed foods are formulated to maximize palatability and are easy to consume in amounts that greatly exceed what the body can process. When concentrated macronutrients (and toxic chemicals) are chronically overconsumed, especially in the context of micronutrient inadequacy and physical inactivity, hormone function and metabolism are disrupted. Mechanisms that evolved to help us meet our energetic needs then become maladaptive and a source of crippling dysfunction.[31] For example, humans evolved to store excess nutrients as fat because it enables survival in times of food scarcity. However, when macronutrient intake continually exceeds energy needs, physiologically normal fat storage progresses to deleterious obesity (see chapter 5).

Metabolic dysfunction begins with a sustained increase in blood glucose and TAG beyond what is needed to meet the body's short- and long-term energy needs. The excess glucose exceeds glycogen storage capacity in the liver and skeletal muscles. Similarly, the combination of excess dietary fat and de novo lipogenesis causes an increase in blood lipids, which exceeds adipose fat storage capacity and promotes adipose cell dysfunction (see chapter 5). When fat storage in adipose tissue is exceeded, the liver, skeletal muscles, kidneys, pancreas, and even the heart also begin to accumulate harmful amounts of ectopic fat, leading to nonalcoholic fatty liver disease (NAFLD) and other metabolic disturbances. The systemic disruption caused by all this excess contributes to insulin resistance, inflammation, metabolic syndrome, and the development of chronic disease.[13,25-28,32-35]

Physical inactivity exacerbates habitual dietary overconsumption because active muscle cells consume large amounts of blood glucose and use stored fat to meet heightened energy needs. Exercise also increases glycogen storage capacity in skeletal muscles; in fact, trained individuals maintain approximately one-third more muscle glycogen than their untrained counterparts. Inactive muscle has reduced energy requirements, which leads to decreased glycogen turnover. As a result, it is unable to support glucose homeostasis.[15]

Diets centered on highly processed foods can also result in micronutrient deficiencies, even when macronutrients are overconsumed. Micronutrients are essential for physiological processes ranging from fat metabolism to DNA transcription, and micronutrient deficiencies increase disease risk.[31] Nutrient supplementation is unlikely the solution: emerging evidence indicates that compensating for micronutrient deficiencies with fortified foods and synthetic vitamins or

What Is Nonalcoholic Fatty Liver Disease?

Nonalcoholic fatty liver disease (NAFLD) is used to describe a range of conditions resulting from excess liver fat and inflammation for reasons other than alcohol use. NAFLD, the most common liver disease worldwide, affects more than 30% of adults and 10% of children in the United States.[53,54] NAFLD is usually diagnosed using liver enzymes, ultrasound, and biopsy, but a score of 30 or greater on the fatty liver index (FLI) was found to be predictive of NAFLD. FLI is also a fairly accurate predictor of insulin resistance and the risk of metabolic syndrome.[55] There are currently no standard treatments or pharmaceuticals specifically designed to treat NAFLD. Although NAFLD can progress into serious liver disease and is associated with cardiometabolic diseases, treatment is not recommended in minor cases without inflammation, most likely because pharmaceutical treatments do not exist. Given that fatty liver increases disease risk and may be one of the first steps toward systemic insulin resistance and inflammation, safe and effective treatments are needed. Data suggest that prolonged water-only fasting may reduce FLI in overweight and obese people.[10]

Fatty Liver Index

The liver is the main regulator of blood glucose, so liver health can be evaluated to assess metabolic health. The FLI uses blood triglycerides (TAGs) and gamma-glutamyl transferase (GGT), body mass index (BMI), and waist circumference to predict incidence of NAFLD and risk of insulin resistance as well as risk of metabolic disease before its development. (Note: GGT is an enzyme that is used to assess liver health.)

FLI values range from 0 to 100; values below 30 rule out fatty liver disease and values above 60 confirm fatty liver disease.

"nutraceuticals" may have deleterious metabolic effects. For example, zinc supplementation can lead to zinc-induced copper deficiency, and multivitamins do not appear to offer any protection from chronic diseases or premature death.[36,37]

We still have a long way to go toward having a complete mechanistic understanding of how macronutrient excess combined with micronutrient deficiency leads to cardiovascular and metabolic diseases. However, there is increasing evidence that systemic insulin resistance and inflammation are primary contributors, and fasting may offer a viable means to reverse these conditions.

Metabolic Syndrome

Metabolic dysfunction results from sustained insulin resistance. It presents clinically as a group of conditions that are highly predictive of future risk of developing chronic diseases.[56] Descriptions of such metabolic dysfunction began to appear in the medical literature around the turn of the 20th century. But names that describe these phenomena, such as metabolic syndrome, syndrome X, and insulin resistance syndrome, did not appear until the 1980s. In the US, people are typically diagnosed with metabolic syndrome according to the criteria of the National Cholesterol Education Program Adult Treatment Panel III, which includes having three of the following conditions:

- increased waist circumference (more than 40 inches in men or 35 inches in women)
- high blood pressure (over 130/85 mmHg)
- high triglyceride (TAG) levels (over 150 mg/dl)
- low high-density lipoprotein (HDL) cholesterol level (less than 40 mg/dl in men or 50 mg/dl in women)
- elevated blood glucose (over 100 mg/dl)

The International Diabetes Federation criteria includes having a large waist circumference plus two more factors. In the US, more than 30% of adults, and more than 50% over the age of 50, have metabolic syndrome.[57] Astonishingly, only 12% of American adults are estimated to be metabolically healthy.[58] Differences in criteria exist worldwide, making it difficult to accurately assess the global prevalence of metabolic syndrome.

The conditions comprising metabolic syndrome often go undiagnosed until chronic disease is established. Excess abdominal fat, typically measured using waist circumference, is particularly damaging because it reflects increased visceral fat, which is highly correlated with insulin resistance. The risk of developing chronic disease also increases with greater levels of visceral fat. Waist circumference is an easily accessible and clear indicator of chronic disease risk.

Fasting Reverses Cardiometabolic Dysfunction

The term *cardiometabolic dysfunction* describes several abnormalities in biomarkers or physical functioning within the cardiovascular and metabolic systems.[38] Many biomarkers used to assess cardiometabolic dysfunction are measured in the blood and influence many of the metabolic processes described previously. Abnormalities in these biomarkers are, with rare exception, indicative of disease development. And although abnormalities often go unnoticed until the later stages of chronic disease, they are usually reversible when identified early. To better diagnose early stage dysfunction, clinicians use validated biomarkers, such as blood lipids and insulin levels, to estimate a person's current state of health and future risk of disease. When values are abnormal, intervention is recommended to revert the values back to a healthy range, which may help avoid infirmity and premature death. If the monitored physiological process is accurately reflected in the biomarkers, and if an intervention safely treats the root cause of the deviation, this can be an effective way to manage health. (See appendix 3 for a detailed description of commonly tested biomarkers.)

We explained earlier how poor diet and physical inactivity contribute to metabolic dysfunction. Dysfunctional glucose and fatty acid metabolism further contribute to vascular dysfunction that can develop into cardiovascular disease. Adopting a health-promoting diet is recommended as a first-line intervention.[39] But most people do not change their diets. Instead, they are prescribed pharmaceuticals in an attempt to correct abnormal biomarkers or symptoms. However, these drugs do not treat the root cause of the abnormality. The fact that up to 70% of American adults chronically use pharmaceutical drugs but more than half remain chronically ill is strong evidence that the current approach is not working.[40,41] There is an urgent need for safe and effective interventions that efficiently improve (or even better, prevent) the underlying causes of cardiometabolic dysfunction. The restorative metabolic processes that occur during prolonged water-only fasting hold potential as one such intervention.

From a purely metabolic perspective, almost nothing is more capable of harnessing the body's innate metabolic capacity to use excess nutrients than consuming only water. Prolonged water-only fasting helps naturally reverse the effects of overconsumption because it removes the source of dietary excess, allowing the body to efficiently use available glucose and glycogen stores. Reduced blood glucose causes a compensatory metabolic switch to increase lipolysis and literally burn through excess fat stores. Sustained fat metabolism during fasting also generates ketones for use in ketosis, which may have additional benefits for health beyond meeting energy requirements.[42,43] One of the most obvious benefits of prolonged water-only fasting is weight loss (see chapter 5). It remains to be determined the extent to which fat loss, increased ketone availability, improved homeostasis, and other physiological changes are responsible for the health improvements that are described in this chapter and throughout this book.

Nonetheless, there have been several published studies demonstrating the potential of prolonged water-only fasting to affect significant changes in cardiometabolic biomarkers.[10,19,30,44-46] The TrueNorth Health Foundation (TNHF) and colleagues have recently published encouraging data on sustained outcomes after prolonged water-only fasting followed by a salt-, oil-, and sugar-free (SOS-free) diet in overweight and obese people.[10,30] Aside from excess weight, they were not in a chronically diseased state, and their pre-fast biomarkers did not indicate active cardiometabolic disease. After an average of two weeks of water-only fasting, there were expected and notable reductions in average body weight, BMI, waist circumference, systolic blood pressure (SBP), and glucose and insulin levels. There were anticipated increases in very low-density lipoprotein (VLDL), triglycerides (TAGs), and high-sensitivity C-reactive protein (hsCRP, a marker of systemic inflammation) as well (see appendix 2). After one week of supervised refeeding, reductions in body weight, BMI, and SBP were sustained from initial post-fast values. Total cholesterol, low-density lipoprotein (LDL) cholesterol (which increased slightly during fasting), and hsCRP (which increased during fasting) all decreased to below pre-fast values. Glucose, insulin, TAGs, and VLDL all increased above pre-fast values as expected, likely due to transient physiological changes in response to the switch from fatty acid metabolism back to glucose metabolism.[30]

To understand the clinical significance of these results, additional data were collected six weeks after supervised refeeding.[10] Body weight, BMI, SBP, total cholesterol, TAGs, LDL cholesterol, hsCRP, glucose, insulin, and gamma-glutamyl transferase (GGT) stabilized at, or continued dropping below, pre-fast levels (see appendixes 2 and 3). TAGs and VLDL decreased between the end of refeeding and follow-up and were within reference ranges but remained above pre-fast levels. There were also slight but potentially meaningful reductions in homeostatic model assessment of insulin resistance (HOMA-IR) and fatty liver index (FLI), which may reduce the risk of metabolic dysfunction. These results demonstrate that many early indicators of cardiometabolic disease improve with a three-week supervised intervention. Furthermore, these changes persisted for at least six weeks, even with imperfect adherence to an SOS-free diet.[10] The degree that diet played in influencing outcomes at six weeks remains unknown and is a necessary focus of future TNHF research. There are more fascinating questions to explore, such as whether repeated fasting would sustain or improve metabolic

FIGURE 4.2. Fasting-induced changes in markers of inflammation and insulin resistance

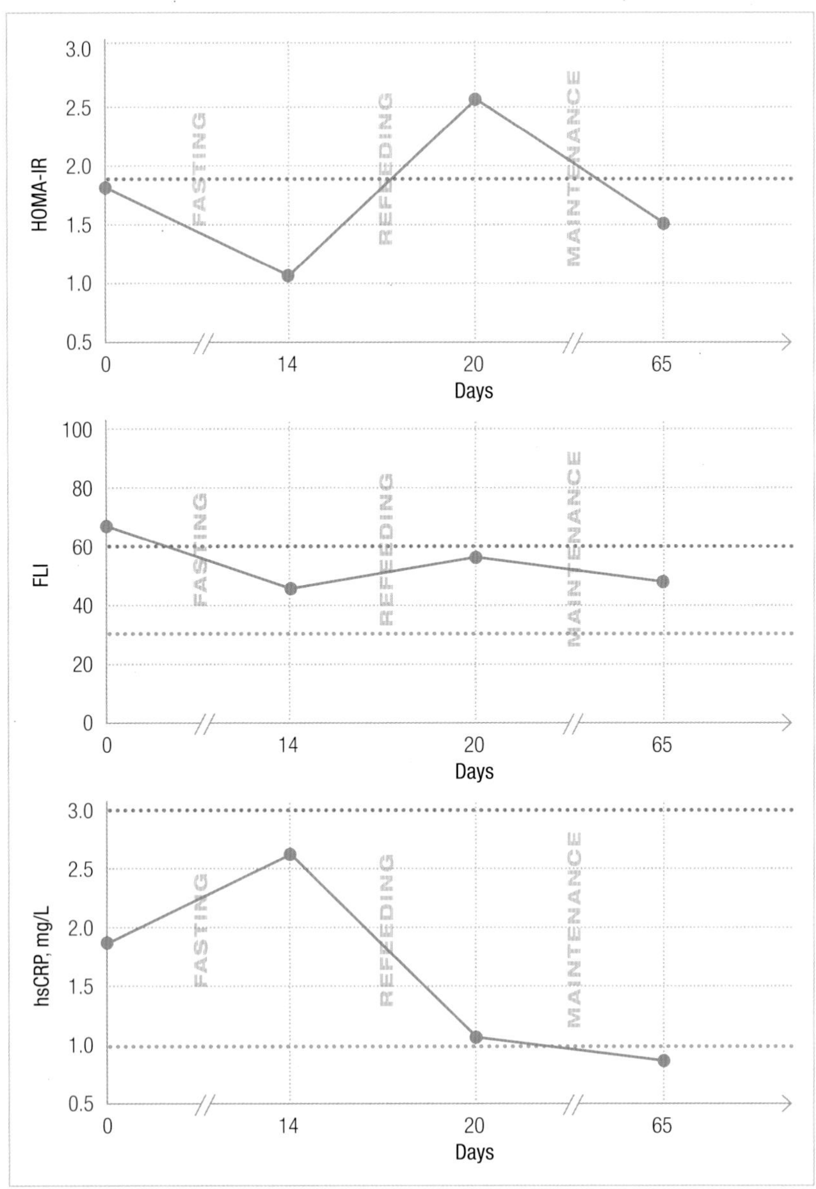

Note: Changes in homeostatic model of assessment of insulin resistance (HOMA-IR), values below 1.9 (red line) indicate optimal insulin sensitivity; fatty liver index (FLI), values 0–30 (green line) are desirable, and values equal to or above 60 (red line) denote the presence of fatty liver disease; high-sensitivity C-reactive protein (hsCRP), values below 1 mg/L (green line) are desirable, and values equal to or above 3 mg/L (red line) denote the presence of inflammation. *N* = 29. Average fasting, refeeding, and maintenance periods were 14, 6, and 45 days, respectively. In the maintenance period, participants were advised to follow a salt-, oil-, and sugar-free diet.[10]

health in this population and if similar results can be quantified in people with metabolic syndrome and type 2 diabetes.

Conclusion

What we eat affects our cellular metabolism, which in turn regulates all our physiological processes. Consuming physiologically normal amounts of nutritious food and getting enough physical activity helps maintain hormonal and metabolic homeostasis. Conversely, overconsumption and inactivity provide a surplus of glucose and fat, increase endogenous glucose and fat production, dysregulate hormones, and lead to metabolic dysfunction. It may be that adherence to a healthy diet and lifestyle is a better predictor of long-term cardiovascular and metabolic health outcomes than any single biomarker. One reason for this is that our cells' response to glucose and insulin is a primary determinant of our overall health. Since poor diet and physical inactivity are primary causes of glucose intolerance and insulin resistance, improving and sustaining metabolic health with diet and physical activity is crucial to managing chronic diseases and supporting healthy aging. It is essential to recognize that chronic disease is not something that happens for no reason or just because we are getting older. Rather, it results from the ways we eat and live. The next chapter will explore obesity, the most visible consequence of metabolic dysfunction.

CASE SUMMARY

Woman has partial regression of unspecified retroperitoneal mass and resolution of enlarged kidney and blocked ureter after prolonged water-only fast followed by an SOS-free diet.

There is a seemingly endless number of physiological abnormalities that appear in the body after prolonged metabolic dysfunction. This is illustrated in our report, published in *Alternative and Complementary Therapies,* of a woman who successfully treated an incidentally identified retroperitoneal mass, hydronephrosis (enlarged kidney), and ureterectasis (blocked ureter) with prolonged water-only fasting and an exclusively whole-plant-food diet free of added salt, oil, and sugar (SOS-free diet).[47] The retroperitoneum is an anatomical region located in the back of the body behind the abdomen. Masses in this region are identified by palpation if they grow big enough, or incidentally with imaging such as MRI and CT scans. More than half of these masses are malignant, and biopsy is regularly indicated. Treatment depends on mass type, location, size, and involvement of nearby organs and includes pharmaceuticals, radiotherapy, chemotherapy, or surgical excision. Ureterectasis, hydronephrosis, and kidney cysts can all block the urinary tract, which may prevent urine flow and require surgical intervention.

A 66-year-old woman arrived at TrueNorth Health Center (TNHC) with the goal of improving her overall health and transitioning to an SOS-free diet. Coincidentally, during the time between her scheduled TNHC visit and her arrival, she was diagnosed with a 4.3 x 4.3 centimeter (cm) unspecified retroperitoneal mass, hydronephrosis, ureterectasis, and kidney cyst and was scheduled for a biopsy 18 days after her medically supervised fasting and refeeding intervention.

Upon the patient's arrival, the fasting supervisor confirmed that the severely obese patient with high blood pressure and normal kidney function could safely water-only fast based on clinical and laboratory examination. She completed 13 days of water-only fasting followed by 11 days of refeeding on an SOS-free diet. While fasting, she reported mild symptoms of nausea, abdominal pain, fatigue, and some chest discomfort on exertion that was carefully assessed by electrocardiogram and clinical monitoring. By the end of the 24-day treatment, she had lost about 7% of her total body weight, and her BMI decreased from 40.6 to 37.9 kg/m^2, bringing her from class 3 (high-risk) to class 2 (moderate-risk) obesity. Her high blood pressure also reached normal levels without the use of antihypertensive medications.

The CT-guided biopsy showed that the retroperitoneal mass had demonstrably reduced to 2.8 x 1.8 cm, and the patient no longer needed to have the mass biopsied. Imaging also revealed total resolution of hydronephrosis and ureterectasis. One year and nine months after the CT scan, the patient reported that she never had a biopsy and did not plan to have another CT scan. She credited continued overall health improvements, including reduced weight and blood pressure, to her healthy diet and lifestyle changes.

Although more follow-up is needed to determine if these health conditions truly resolved, this case sets a precedent for additional research into the use of water-only fasting and whole-plant-food diets as low-risk, interim treatments for the management of retroperitoneal masses while the patient awaits full diagnosis via biopsy.

CHAPTER 5

Fasting Reverses Obesity

Chronic (or noncommunicable) diseases are usually thought to be incurable, may get worse over time or limit daily activities, and require ongoing medical management.[1] Worldwide, more than 3 billion adults have one or more chronic diseases. In the US, 6 out of 10, or more than 150 million adults, have one or more chronic diseases, increasing to 8 out of 10 adults over age 65.[2] Of the 10 most common causes of death in the US, more than half are chronic diseases, and nearly 80% of all deaths are caused by just five chronic diseases.[3]

Chronic diseases are also the leading cause of death globally, resulting in more than 40 million deaths annually.[4] This is more than double the number of deaths from infectious diseases, maternal and perinatal disorders, and nutritional deficiencies combined.[5] More and more people are living with the costly burden of both chronic and infectious diseases. This is especially concerning because recent pandemics have established that the chronically ill may be more susceptible to infectious diseases, experience deleterious immune responses, and have higher death rates.[6] For example, people under 40 who have three or more chronic diseases are more than 15 times more likely to die from COVID-19 compared to healthy people, with more than half of COVID-19 deaths attributable to chronic disease.[7]

The economic effects are also devastating. In 2022, the estimated annual healthcare costs for chronic disease in the US exceeded $3.5 trillion, more than 40% higher than costs in other economically developed countries.[2,8] People in the US, however, are among the least healthy worldwide. This paradox is driven primarily by the fact that in the US, poor health results from the overconsumption of highly processed food combined with physical inactivity and drug use, not a lack of medical care or pharmaceutical drug use.

TABLE 5.1. **Prevalence of chronic disease among most common causes of death in the US**

	CAUSE	DEATHS PER YEAR, *N*	% OF TOTAL DEATHS	PREVALENCE OF CHRONIC DISEASE, *N* (%)
		2,094,893	100	
1	Heart diseases	655,381	23	127,900,000 (38.1)
2	Cancer	599,274	21	5-year prevalent cases: 8,432,938 (2.5)
3	Accidents	167,127	6	
4	Chronic lower respiratory diseases	159,486	6	12,500,000 (3.7)
5	Cerebrovascular disease	147,810	5	
6	Alzheimer's disease	122,019	4	5,800,000 (1.7)
7	Diabetes mellitus	84,946	3	37,300,000 (11.2)
8	Influenza and pneumonia	59,120	2	
9	Kidney disease	51,386	2	37,000,000 (11.0)
10	Suicide	48,344	2	

Table data sources: See references 3, 69-78. Note: Ten most common causes of death and prevalence of chronic disease in the US, 2019–2021.

Highly processed foods, which are low in nutrients, high in calories, and full of chemicals, were rarely eaten before the 1950s.[9,10] Now, more than half of all food consumed in the US is highly processed.[11] In just 75 years, this synthetic food group has become the most commonly consumed, with the majority of people eating far more of it than whole and less processed foods found in nature. It is astonishing that something so harmful can be manufactured and consumed in such copious amounts. One explanation is that these foods are designed to electrify our taste buds, coaxing us into a pleasure trap that overrides our natural impulse to eat physiologically healthy amounts of food. From this perspective, it is challenging to put responsibility entirely on an individual's free will when companies producing the food deliberately design it so that you will not want to stop eating. This explains why highly processed foods continue to be manufactured in such large amounts: their production is highly profitable. The global vegetable oil market alone, for example, is estimated at $100 billion per year.[12]

Despite the irrefutable link between increased consumption of highly processed foods and high rates of obesity and other chronic

TABLE 5.2. **Comparison of pharma revenue versus total healthcare expenditure versus chronic disease rates in US**

YEAR	ANNUAL REVENUE OF US PHARMA INDUSTRY, IN BILLIONS	NATIONAL HEALTHCARE EXPENDITURE, IN BILLIONS	CHRONIC DISEASE RATES
2010	291	2,589.6	45%
2015	302	3,165.4	53%
2020	424	4,144.1	62.6%

Table data sources: See references 13, 79, 80. Values based on available information. Note: Chronic disease rates are the percentage of total population with at least one chronic disease.

diseases, the problem snowballs year after year. This connection underscores the reality that most people do not become obese or chronically ill due to genetics or a simple lack of willpower. It is clear that unhealthful eating causes massive, measurable problems. Discouragingly, there have been very few policy-based or patient-oriented approaches aimed at ameliorating this health crisis. This is likely because food, pharmaceutical, and medical enterprises are making record-breaking profits.[13-16]

Obesity

Obesity is the most visible consequence of overeating and greatly increases the risk of developing chronic diseases. Overweight and obesity are defined as excess fat mass, which is typically measured using the body mass index (BMI).[17] Obesity is largely due to excess subcutaneous fat, located beneath the skin surface. Most obese people also have excess visceral fat, which accumulates around organs in the abdominal area and can be highly inflammatory.[18] Research suggests that the risks associated with obesity may have more to do with excess visceral fat than the more abundant subcutaneous fat, which may actually be protective as suggested by improved glucose tolerance and insulin sensitivity in animal models.[19] An increasing number of "normal-weight" people are actually metabolically unhealthy, most likely due, in part, to excess visceral fat.[20,21] Currently in the US, more than 70% of adults are overweight. Of those, more than 40% are classified as obese, and at least 10% of those are classified as severely obese. Even more alarmingly, nearly 40% of school-age children are now overweight or obese.[22]

The Centers for Disease Control and Prevention reports that the increasing rates of obesity began in the 1980s.[23] National anthropo-

TABLE 5.3. **BMI categories and US and global obesity prevalence in 2020**

WEIGHT CATEGORIES		PREVALENCE, %	
	BMI, kg/m^2	US	Global
Underweight	< 18.50	2	9
Normal weight	18.50–24.99	25	52
Overweight	≥ 25–29	31	26
Obesity	≥ 30	42	13

Table data sources: See references 17, 23. Note: Prevalence rates as determined from available information. Body mass index (BMI) is calculated using weight and height (kg/m^2).[81] It is used in clinical settings to determine risk and treatment plans. It is used in research settings to facilitate categorization and discovery. Importantly, BMI alone does not reveal the extent to which a person's body mass is composed of lean muscle or fat, whether the fat is stored subcutaneously or viscerally, or if the individual is metabolically healthy. For example, 5% to 45% of people who have a normal weight are considered metabolically unhealthy, and approximately 5% of people who are obese are considered metabolically healthy.[20]

FIGURE 5.1. **Dual-energy x-ray absorptiometry scans showing the body composition of normal-weight, overweight, and obese people**

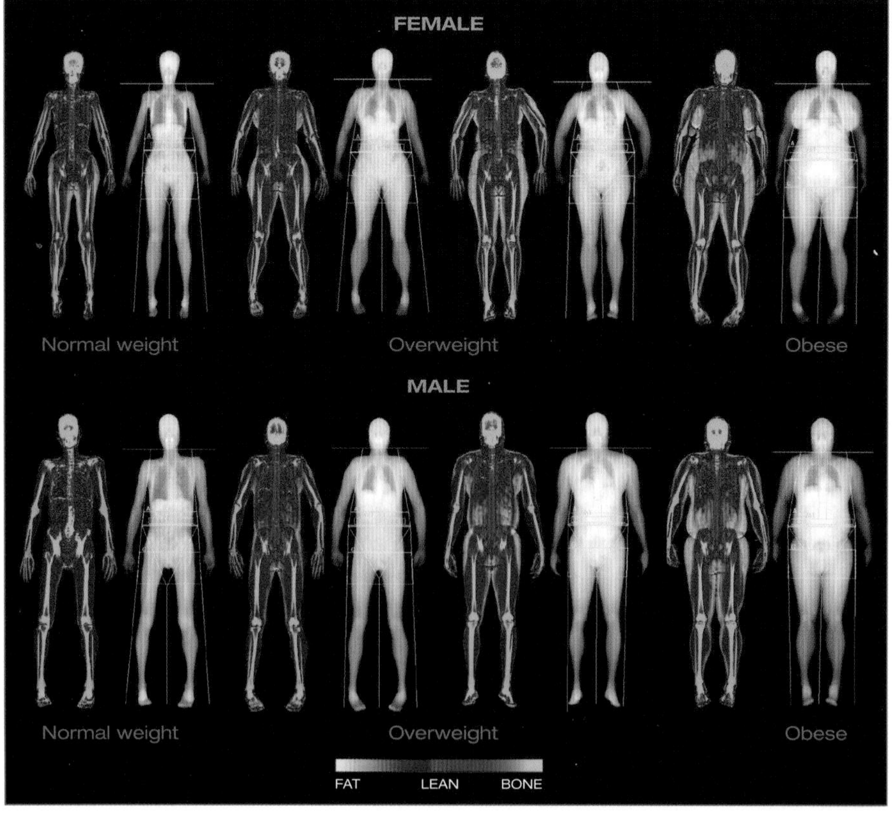

metric data indicate that, in 1980, only 15% of American adults were classified as obese. However, birth cohorts from 1882 to 1986 indicate that Americans have been steadily gaining weight for more than 100 years, with two notable accelerations in average BMI. The first uptick began after World War I in the 1920s and lasted through the 1940s, and the second began after World War II in the 1950s and persists to this day.[24] The growth after World War I mostly occurred in the lower BMI categories, and rates of obesity were negligible. In contrast, after World War II, consistent growth has occurred in upper BMI categories, with the highest category increasing 10% to 30%, depending on the population. Furthermore, people born after 1950 experience much higher rates of obesity than those born before.[24] Notably, the rapid increase in BMI after World War II coincided with a period marked by significant postindustrial lifestyle changes including increased television viewing, prevalent automobile use, and, most importantly, consumption of highly processed and fast food.

Rates of overweight and obesity in people of all ages are increasing globally.[25,26] In fact, the decline of a country from lean to obese is so common and follows such a predictable pattern that it has been characterized into distinct stages.[27] The first stage is characterized by increasing rates of obesity in women of higher socioeconomic status. The second stage is reflected by increased rates of obesity in all adults and children, with a narrowing gap between members of higher and lower socioeconomic classes. The third and final stage occurs when rates of obesity in adults with lower socioeconomic status surpass those with higher socioeconomic status. What's more, no nation is immune to this transformation. In 2016, Vietnam was reportedly the only country to maintain obesity rates below 5%, but obesity rates are now on the rise there as well.[27] This paints a troubling picture for the future of global health because obesity correlates with the development of metabolic syndrome and associated chronic diseases including cardiovascular disease, type 2 diabetes, and certain cancers.[28] Obesity is also among the leading causes of preventable premature death.

Why Are Humans So Prone to Obesity?

Obesity pathogenesis begins with sustained overconsumption—typically of foods that are high in calories and low in nutrients—paired with decreased physical activity, which leads to caloric intake in excess of energy expenditure.[28,29] It is historically accepted that, in terms of weight gain, a calorie is a calorie. However, it may not be as simple as "calories in, calories out" because not only are people consuming more calories, but their calories are coming from highly processed foods containing unnatural amounts of sugar, oil, and salt. These calories are accompanied by nonnutritive chemicals, which are highly palatable (and therefore habitually overconsumed) and also adversely affect our metabolism and contribute to related morbidities.[30,31] A study comparing two weeks on an unrestricted ultraprocessed food diet with an unprocessed food diet found that people who consumed ultraprocessed foods ate more calories and gained weight while people who ate unprocessed foods consumed fewer calories and lost weight.[32] Although it is technically possible to become obese eating minimally processed whole foods, it is rare because of an insufficient drive to habitually overeat these foods. Also, minimally processed whole foods do not usually contain substances such as obesogenic chemicals (e.g., the plasticizer BPA and the insecticide DDT) that adversely affect metabolism and cause weight gain.[33] In addition to endocrine-disrupting chemicals, several genetic mutations and epigenetic modifications have been identified as contributing to the onset of obesity,[34] but the primary factor driving the obesity pandemic appears to be the habitual overconsumption of highly processed foods.

Some scientists say that the second step in obesity pathogenesis involves the "biological defense" to hold on to excess fat.[35] This may happen because, throughout human evolution, opportunities to overconsume calorically dense foods were rare. It is plausible that such foods were overeaten when they became available and that excess calories were stored as fat to ensure survival when food was scarce or during illness. Each person may have a different range of upper and lower weight set points based on their genetic or epigenetic makeup. Some people may have an upper set point high enough to allow them to overeat until they become obese, especially when exposed to a continuous supply of cheap, tasty, highly processed foods. At that point, their physiological response is to maintain this increased weight through mechanisms that stimulate or suppress the drive to eat and the ability to store or metabolize fat.

As mentioned earlier, fat can be stored viscerally or subcutaneously. One explanation for excess accumulation of visceral fat—even in the absence of excess subcutaneous fat—involves the concept of a personal fat threshold.[36] This theory suggests that individuals have variable capacities to store subcutaneous fat. Once the subcutaneous fat threshold is reached, additional body fat is stored viscerally and ectopically in the liver, pancreas, and heart and skeletal muscles. Someone with a high personal fat threshold can therefore become overweight or obese with excess subcutaneous fat without being metabolically unhealthy because they have not accumulated large amounts of harmful visceral fat. Conversely, a person with a low personal fat threshold is unable to accumulate large amounts of subcutaneous fat stores and therefore accumulates large stores of detrimental visceral fat. This, in turn, can lead to metabolic dysfunction, even at a normal body weight. It should be noted that, if dietary habits are not improved, nearly all metabolically healthy overweight individuals will eventually surpass their personal fat threshold and become metabolically unhealthy. Encouragingly, once weight loss is initiated in metabolically unhealthy, obese individuals, markers of metabolic health improve long before normal weight is achieved.[37] This suggests that clinically meaningful visceral fat loss is prioritized and occurs before subcutaneous fat stores diminish significantly. We will present research later in this chapter that demonstrates this beneficial biological phenomenon.

Excess Visceral Fat Wreaks Metabolic Havoc

Visceral fat is located deep in the abdominal area around our organs. Excess visceral fat is associated with increased risk of metabolic syndrome, regardless of obesity status.[38] Blood glucose and lipid levels are normally maintained within a tight physiological range, and excess sugar and fat are burned or stored to maintain this balance. If excessive caloric consumption continues and physical activity is minimal, the body must deposit this surplus. Subcutaneous fat stores expand, and visceral fat cells begin to enlarge (hypertrophy). If these cells grow to their maximal size, the continued caloric surplus drives the cell population to expand through dysregulated proliferation (hyperplasia). In other words, the fat cells divide and multiply. Visceral fat cells are dysfunctional in that they demonstrate an impaired response to insulin, diminished glucose uptake, and blunted fatty acid metabolism. Eventually, they will become insulin resistant.[39] These cells also produce harmful quantities of inflammatory proteins (adipokines) and lipotoxins.[40] This imbalance contributes to local and systemic inflammation through several complex (and seemingly protective) mechanisms, which have mostly been studied in animal models.[39,41] The effects of this process can be devastating: sustained inflammation appears to be involved in the progression of essentially all chronic diseases.[42,43]

This type of dysfunction is a classic example of how natural physiological processes that evolved to enhance survival can become pathological when environmental factors are out of balance. Despite prolific research, the physiological mechanisms that interact to regulate this process (e.g., neuroendocrine pathways and signaling in the gut-brain axis) remain poorly understood.[44,45] Fortunately, we do not need to know exactly why humans are prone to obesity, nor do we need to understand all the physiological details in order to see that lifestyle interventions such as prolonged water-only fasting effectively reverse obesity, reduce excess visceral fat, and lower biomarkers of systemic inflammation.

Prolonged Water-Only Fasting Reverses Obesity

Sustained weight loss of just 5% of one's body weight produces clinically significant reductions in disease risk.[37] Unfortunately, most weight-loss interventions, aside from diet and lifestyle, have proven neither safe nor effective.[46] Furthermore, most people do not sufficiently adhere to a healthy diet to prevent or reverse obesity.[47] Prolonged water-only fasting may constitute a uniquely valuable intervention for preventing and reducing obesity because some evidence indicates that fasting modulates taste sensitivity and increases enjoyment and consumption of whole-plant foods while decreasing preference for sweet, salty, and fatty foods.[48] This is important because the hedonistic response to highly processed food impedes the willingness to make and sustain healthy changes.

Prolonged water-only fasting has been used as a weight-loss treatment for obesity since around 1960, when rates of obesity were only 13%.[49] Reports published in the scientific literature from this period demonstrate that prolonged water-only fasting is among the most effective weight-loss strategies, with an estimated initial loss of about 2 pounds per day and a gradual reduction and stabilization at about 0.7 pounds per day over 30 days of fasting.[50] Prolonged water-only fasting was eventually abandoned as an obesity treatment because of the harmful fasting practices used during this time (see chapter 2).[51] Fortunately, the latest research has consistently demonstrated that, with current protocols and expert medical supervision, appropriate candidates can safely practice prolonged water-only fasting for up to 40 days.[52,53]

Recent studies report weight loss of similar magnitudes to those reported in earlier research.[48,54-56] People are reported to lose an average of 11% of their total body weight after approximately two weeks of fasting, which is substantially greater than the 5% loss established to reduce disease risk. Fasting also accomplishes this feat in a much shorter time span than other weight-loss methods that produce similar results.[55,57] The value of weight loss, however, can be limited by the impending weight regain that often follows many interventions. In the case of prolonged water-only fasting, only 2% of total body weight was regained after approximately five days of controlled refeeding, and weight loss was maintained for at least six weeks after the fasting and refeeding intervention, with imperfect adherence to dietary recommendations.[56,57] Regaining weight is common with most weight-loss methods: a meta-analysis found that 50% of people regain all the weight lost within two years.[58] Remarkably, in another TrueNorth Health Foundation (TNHF) study, nearly 75% of the people who were obese at the start had maintained their weight loss or continued losing weight for up to one year, and the others had not gained weight beyond their starting weight.[56] Additional research is necessary to validate these findings, but it is also notable that 40% of obese people moved into the overweight category, and 54% of overweight people moved into the normal-weight category. This suggests that repeated fasting could incrementally help people with obesity achieve normal weight and, perhaps more importantly, help overweight people avoid obesity in the first place.

Although these studies were conducted in a unique population with an interest in fasting, the data reveal that weight loss can persist for at least six weeks, and in some cases one year, after the prolonged water-only fast. These results are extremely encouraging, in part because they begin to dispel the popular criticism that weight lost during prolonged water-only fasting is not sustained and may rebound above the starting weight.[59] This criticism has been used as justification against the therapeutic use of prolonged water-only fasting for fat loss.[60] However, these promising results indicate that fasting efficiently produces clinically meaningful and sustainable reductions in body weight and body fat, and they underscore that, once a person corrects the diet and lifestyle choices that initially triggered their weight gain, maintaining fasting-induced weight loss becomes possible.

Larger studies with long-term follow-up visits are needed to determine rates of sustained weight loss in the general population. Moreover, patient-centered research is needed to better treat obesity. For example, the average length of a medically supervised water-only fast at TrueNorth Health Center (TNHC) is about one to two weeks, and fasts up to

FIGURE 5.2. **Fasting-induced changes in body composition**

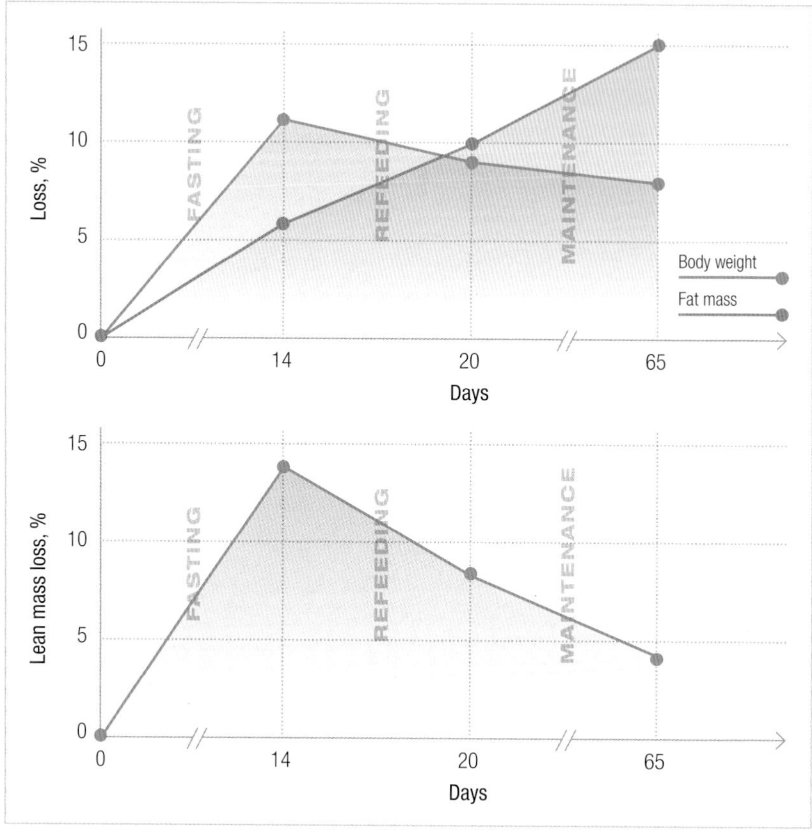

Note: Percentage loss of total body weight and fat mass and lean and fat mass during average fasting, refeeding, and maintenance periods of 14, 6, and 45 days, respectively. In the maintenance period, participants were advised to follow a salt-, oil-, and sugar-free diet.[56,57]

40 consecutive days are infrequent. In the research presented here, fasts ranged from 10 to 40 days, but it is unknown whether longer fasts are more effective than shorter fasts. Furthermore, repeated fasting with a sufficiently restorative intervening period may be required to normalize body weight. As is commonplace to all lines of scientific inquiry, several uncertainties remain, but these preliminary weight-loss data indicate that prolonged water-only fasting produces similar or better results than the most effective pharmaceutical interventions and intermittent fasting methods.[46,61,62] This method holds additional promise, considering that prolonged water-only fasting may also increase acceptance of and adherence to a health-promoting diet, potentially setting the stage for more desirable long-term outcomes.[48]

Fat Loss Continues Even after Fasting Ends

The significant weight loss that occurs during fasting is well established, but less is known about how body composition (i.e., amounts of fat, lean, and bone mass) changes. One way this question has been addressed is by using dual-energy x-ray absorptiometry (DXA) scans to measure body composition before and after fasting.[63] Note that DXA scans are limited by their inability to distinguish whether lean mass loss results from muscle protein or the large amounts of glycogen (stored glucose) and accompanying fluid found within the muscle. This is important because reductions in muscle protein may have more detrimental consequences and require more time to rebuild, whereas glycogen and fluid repletion can occur quickly and easily with refeeding on a whole-food diet. Nonetheless, DXA is one of the safest and most accessible means to assess body composition today.

Research into changes in body composition conducted at TNHF found an interesting pattern of weight loss in overweight and obese people, especially regarding fat loss.[56] After approximately two weeks of fasting, people lost an average of 6% of their total fat mass, which accounted for about 25% of the total body weight lost. After about six days of controlled refeeding, total body weight increased by 2%, but average total fat mass continued to decrease for an average total loss of 10%. Total lean mass rapidly increased with food reintroduction in all populations.[57,64,65] Fat loss continued and six weeks later, average total fat mass lost was 15%, which accounted for about 75% of the total body weight lost. Remarkably, there is also a substantial amount of additional visceral fat loss after fasting ends. Visceral fat loss may contribute to the overall improvements observed in cardiovascular, metabolic, and inflammatory biomarkers (see chapter 4). A similar fat loss pattern is observed in normal-weight male and female volunteers, suggesting that prolonged water-only fasting may be an effective way to prevent unwanted (and seemingly inevitable) visceral fat gain over a lifetime.[56,64,65]

Conclusion

We are in the middle of a major public health crisis of obesity and other chronic diseases. Although these afflictions are often treated as independent pathologies, all result primarily from dysfunctional metabolism caused by the overconsumption of highly processed foods. A more

FIGURE 5.3. Fasting-induced changes in visceral fat mass

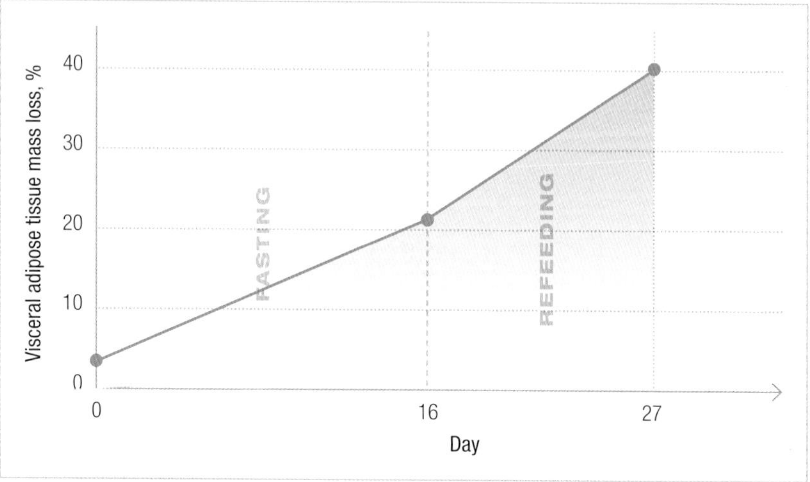

Note: Average percentage visceral adipose tissue mass loss in three healthy men while fasting and refeeding. The fasting period averaged 16 days and the refeeding period averaged 11 days.

integrated understanding of the human body recognizes that these conditions are interrelated, and that our innate physiological intelligence can naturally restore our health when we replace unhealthful behaviors with healthful ones. A rolling succession of medical professionals, nutrition experts, and wellness gurus offer dietary advice that frequently improves health, at least in some people, for some amount of time, but not because the fad diets they promote are backed by meaningful evidence that supports their health claims. On the contrary, their core tenets are typically scientifically ungrounded. Rather, these diets occasionally improve body weight and overall health because they recommend eating more whole foods and fewer highly processed foods. Thus, it seems that regardless of what specific whole foods are being consumed, simply eating fewer highly processed foods goes a long way toward improving health outcomes.

Ultimately, this is great news because it means that simple, straightforward diet and lifestyle changes can lead to significant and lasting improvements in quality of life. This is easier said than done, however, because we are now more disconnected from natural food and healthy lifestyle practices than ever before, and most people are ill-equipped to change without support. Thankfully, prolonged water-only fasting is a powerful tool that may remedy unproductive behaviors and begin to reverse the consequences of overconsumption. In particular, prolonged water-only fasting demonstrates exceptional potential as a treatment not only for reducing weight but also for adopting health-promoting habits. Considering that the rate of obesity has steadily risen to more than 40% in American adults and that obesity increases the risk of developing type 2 diabetes, hypertension, dyslipidemia, and other chronic diseases, it follows that fasting may also reduce chronic disease rates. Only research with a sufficiently large population followed for a sufficient length of time can confirm such effects, but there is evidence that prolonged water-only fasting does more than just reduce weight; it also effectively reduces high blood pressure, which is the leading preventable factor for cardiovascular disease and all-cause mortality worldwide.[66,67]

CASE SUMMARY

Visceral fat loss is greater in normal-weight men during and after prolonged water-only fasting.

As we mentioned, excess visceral fat (visceral adipose tissue, VAT) increases biomarkers of systemic inflammation and is strongly associated with cardiovascular and metabolic diseases—even in individuals of otherwise normal weight. All weight-loss methods seem to reduce visceral fat to some extent, but very low-calorie ketogenic diets reportedly do so more rapidly than others.[68] In our case series published in the *International Journal of Disease Reversal and Prevention*, we reported on the body composition changes in three normal-weight men who completed a prolonged water-only fast followed by an exclusively whole-plant-food diet free of added salt, oil, and sugar (SOS-free diet).[65]

Body composition was measured using DXA before fasting, upon completion of fasting, and after completion of refeeding.

The first patient was a 27-year-old man who fasted for 15 days and followed the fast with a refeed of 6 days. By the end of refeeding, he had lost 17.4 pounds (10%) of total body weight, 7.7 pounds (17%) of total fat, 0.5 pound (54%) of total VAT, and 9.6 pounds (8%) of total lean mass. Notably, 5 pounds (33%) of lean mass lost during fasting was regained by the end of refeeding.

The second patient was a 38-year-old male who fasted for 14 days and followed the fast with a refeed of 15 days. By the end of refeeding, he had lost 9.9 pounds (6%) of total body weight, 6.0 pounds (15%) of total fat, 0.6 pound (41%) of total VAT, and 4.0 pounds (4%) of total lean mass. Notably, 8 pounds (67%) of the lean mass lost during fasting was regained by the end of refeeding (see table 5.4).

The third patient was a 40-year-old male who fasted for 20 days and followed the fast with a refeed of 11 days. By the end of his refeeding, he had lost 19.0 pounds (10%) of total body weight, 9.3 pounds (22%) of total fat, 0.3 pound (24%) of total VAT, and 9.7 pounds (7%) of total lean mass. Notably, 6 pounds (38%) of the lean mass lost during fasting was regained by the end of refeeding (see table 5.4).

Although all three patients were normal weight, all had excess abdominal fat and lost more than 20% of their visceral fat by the end of fasting. Substantial visceral fat loss continued even after food reintroduction despite increases in total body weight during the same period. The role that diet played in this continued visceral fat loss is unknown.

Finally, it remains unclear whether changes in lean mass throughout fasting and refeeding were due to fluctuations in proteins, glycogen (localized energy storage in muscle and other organs), or fluid. Lean mass initially decreased but partially returned after refeeding, even without resistance exercise (e.g., weight lifting), which suggests that most changes in lean mass were due to depletion and repletion of glycogen and the accompanying fluid.

TABLE 5.4. **Changes in body composition in normal-weight men after fasting**

	STAGE OF FASTING	BMI (kg/m^2)	TOTAL MASS (lb)	LEAN MASS (lb)	TOTAL FAT (lb)	TOTAL VAT MASS (lb)
Case 1	SOF (day 0)	24	179	125	46	0.89
	EOF (day 15)	21	159	110	41	0.64
	EOR (day 21)	22	161	115	39	0.41
Case 2	SOF (day 0)	23	158	111	40	1.41
	EOF (day 14)	21	141	99	36	1.10
	EOR (day 29)	21	147	107	34	0.83
Case 3	SOF (day 0)	25	188	140	42	1.06
	EOF (day 20)	22	165	124	35	0.90
	EOR (day 31)	22	169	130	33	0.81

Note: BMI, body mass index; EOF, end of fast; EOR, end of refeeding; kg, kilogram; lb, pound; m, meter; SOF, start of fast.

CHAPTER 6

Fasting Reverses Hypertension

Another area where prolonged water-only fasting holds tremendous lifesaving potential is the treatment of high blood pressure. High blood pressure, or hypertension, is extremely prevalent and increases the risk of several diseases as well as death from all causes, yet common treatment options frequently fall short. Fasting, on the other hand, consistently normalizes blood pressure, even in people with severe hypertension. In this chapter, we will detail the latest and most robust clinical evidence indicating that fasting effectively reduces blood pressure. Recent research has also begun to address long-standing questions about the sustainability of health benefits gained while water-only fasting. Indeed, data indicate that of the participants who provided follow-up data, most sustained their fasting-induced blood pressure reductions and other outcomes for at least one year.[1] The promising results have spurred more research, which is currently underway and may establish that medically supervised prolonged water-only fasting is a superior intervention for stage 1 and stage 2 hypertension. These types of studies are notable: historically it has been difficult to research or publish findings because prolonged water-only fasting has long been stigmatized. In this chapter, we will explain the complexities, limitations, and obstacles that clinicians and scientists face when attempting to establish fasting as a treatment option for hypertension.

Hypertension

Blood pressure is the amount of force that blood applies against our arteries as it flows throughout the body. Our heartbeat produces the force to pump blood and generate blood pressure, which is measured

TABLE 6.1. **Hypertension classification**

BP CATEGORY	SBP, mmHg		DBP, mmHg
Normal	< 120	and	< 80
Prehypertension	120 to 129	and	80 to 89
Stage 1 HTN	130 to 139	or	80 to 89
Stage 2 HTN	≥ 140	or	≥ 90

Table data source: See reference 30. Note: BP, blood pressure; DBP, diastolic blood pressure; HTN, hypertension; mmHg, millimeters of mercury; SBP, systolic blood pressure.

in millimeters of mercury (mmHg). Systolic blood pressure (SBP) is the maximum amount of pressure exerted when the heart pumps, and diastolic blood pressure (DBP) is the maximum amount of pressure exerted when the heart relaxes between contractions. Blood pressure, like body weight, has been identified as a cardiometabolic biomarker that can chronically elevate and develop into debilitating disease. When blood pressure is consistently high, it can lead to hardening of the arteries, kidney disease, stroke, and an array of other disorders.

Hypertension is defined as having consecutive systolic/diastolic blood pressure (SBP/DBP) readings of 130/80 mmHg or higher. Globally, more than one billion adults have hypertension, and it is the leading cause of death and disability.[2,3] In the US, 120 million adults (nearly 50%) have hypertension, and an additional 30% are estimated to have prehypertension (120 to 129/80 to 89 mmHg).[4,5] High blood pressure is frequently asymptomatic, and approximately 36% of people go undiagnosed. Among those who are diagnosed, more than half are unable to adequately control their blood pressure with antihypertensive medication.[6,7] Uncontrolled hypertension is a major risk factor for cardiovascular disease and stroke and contributes to more than 400,000 deaths per year in the US alone. The burden to the US economy is also massive: nearly $200 billion annually and rising.[8,9]

These statistics are staggering considering it is widely known that unhealthy diet and lifestyle choices are leading contributors to high blood pressure.[10] And although diet and lifestyle changes are encouraged as preventative strategies, the standard in US medical care is to prescribe antihypertensive medications instead of dealing with the reasons that cause high blood pressure in the first place. Unfortunately, the data show that antihypertensive medications yield only modest reductions in blood pressure and do not significantly lower associated health risks.[11,12] These medications also come with the significant risk of multiple side effects, which increase with more intensive or combination treatments that are typically required to meaningfully lower blood pressure.[13] Furthermore, approximately 45% of patients do not adhere to prescribed medications for various reasons, including side effects.[14-16] These statistics suggest that current treatment strategies are inadequate.

We know that hypertension is correlated with various lifestyle factors, including tobacco use, processed diet, excessive alcohol consumption, physical inactivity, high stress, and various chronic conditions. However, there is a lack of robust data on the effect of lifestyle change, including diet, on blood pressure and associated cardiovascular disease outcomes.[10] The most reliable data come from Dietary Approaches to Stop Hypertension (DASH) research, but DASH dietary interventions reduced SBP/DBP by an average of only 5.2/2.6 mmHg,[17] which is less effective than other dietary approaches.[34-36] For example, a small study found that completing a prolonged, very low-calorie liquid diet followed by a three-month DASH diet lowered blood pressure more effectively than the DASH diet alone.[18] Considering that sufficiently lowering high blood pressure has the potential to reduce all-cause mortality, it is imperative that more effective treatments are established.

Prolonged water-only fasting reduces blood pressure in everyone who fasts—although the value almost never falls below normal range, even in normotensive people, except transiently as indicated by reports of presyncope upon standing while fasting (see chapter 3). The observation that fasting lowers blood pressure led to the use of prolonged water-only fasting to treat people with hypertension. Several research studies have quantified these effects, and substantial data from multiple studies indicate that prolonged water-only fasting followed by an exclusively whole-plant-food diet free of salt, oil, and sugar (SOS-free diet) reduces high blood pressure. In 2001 and 2002, after decades of observing outstanding results in hypertensive patients who undertook fasts, Dr. Goldhamer and colleagues published two retrospective studies showing remarkable reductions in blood pressure. In one study, in 68 consecutive patients with borderline high blood pressure, 13 days of water-only fasting reduced SBP by 20 mmHg on average, with 82% of patients achieving SBP below 120 mmHg.[19] In a second study of 174 consecutive patients with high blood pressure, an average of 10 days of water-only fasting resulted in more than 90% of patients becoming normotensive. In patients with SBP greater than 140 mmHg, the average reduction in SBP was 37 mmHg, and reductions were even greater in patients with SBP exceeding 160 mmHg.[20] Although widely acknowledged, these studies have been justifiably criticized as inconclusive due to limitations inherent to retrospective data collection and a lack of follow-up research. Nevertheless, they provide intriguing preliminary evidence that medically supervised prolonged water-only fasting may offer promise as a potential treatment of hypertension.

Current Evidence That Fasting Lowers High Blood Pressure

Taking steps toward validating the effects of fasting on blood pressure, TrueNorth Health Foundation (TNHF) recently conducted a prospective study investigating the safety and feasibility of medically supervised prolonged water-only fasting in the treatment of stage 1 and stage 2 hypertension.[1] This study is the first to closely monitor adverse events and assess treatment adherence and acceptance, specifically in a hypertensive population. The 29 participants included people with stage 1 and stage 2 hypertension. The fasting period ranged from 7 to 40 days, with an average fast length of 11 days. This was followed by an average of 5 days of supervised, stepwise refeeding on an SOS-free diet. Notably, all people taking antihypertensive medications were completely weaned off medications before fasting.

As expected, we observed clinically meaningful reductions in blood pressure. At baseline, the participants' average blood pressure was 147/86 mmHg, which dropped to 113/77 mmHg by the end of refeeding. Reductions were even greater in people with stage 2 hypertension at baseline: this group had an average blood pressure of 158/90 mmHg, which dropped to 115/80 mmHg by the end of refeeding. These data indicate that fewer than two weeks of fasting and refeeding efficiently reduce blood pressure, validating previously published data and fasting clinicians' common knowledge. This study also addressed the sustainability of reductions in blood pressure, which is critical to determining the clinical utility of treatment. To explore this issue, blood pressure was measured six weeks after the supervised refeeding period. The average blood pressure after six weeks increased only slightly, from 115/80 mmHg to 122/76 mmHg. Even people with stage 2 hypertension at baseline maintained an average blood pressure of 125/78 mmHg for at least six weeks—and without medication! Of the five people who were taking antihypertensive medications at baseline, only one had resumed medication (at half of the baseline dose) after six weeks (see appendix 4).

Self-reported adherence to the recommended SOS-free diet was only slightly better than before fasting, and the role of diet in maintaining blood pressure reductions induced by water-only fasting remains to be determined. Furthermore, most reported adverse events, such as fatigue and nausea, were mild to moderate. These data aligned with the retrospective adverse event data[21] (see chapter 3), and the laboratory results included in the analysis expanded our understanding. There were no unexpected, serious, or sustained adverse events. Adherence to the treatment protocol exceeded 90%, and most participants

FIGURE 6.1. Reductions in blood pressure

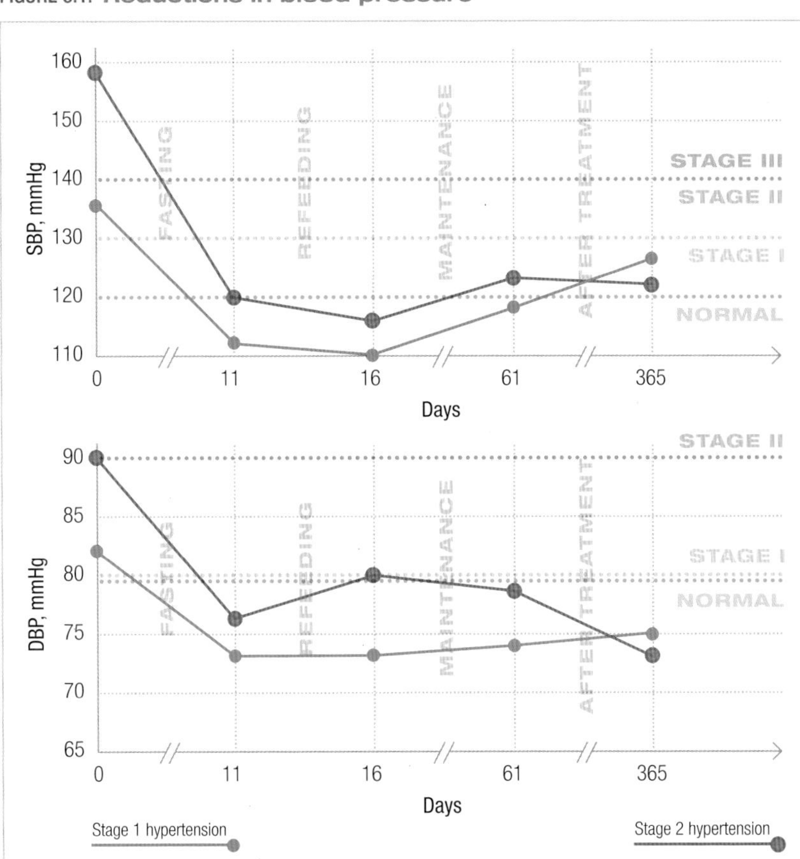

Note: Changes in systolic blood pressure (SBP) and diastolic blood pressure (DBP) in people with stage 1 (blue) and stage 2 (red) hypertension. The average fasting, refeeding, and maintenance periods were 11, 5, and 45 days, respectively. Data were also collected after one year.[1]

reported that the treatment was highly acceptable and preferable to pharmaceutical therapy.

Approximately one year after the fasting and refeeding intervention, data were collected from 17 of the original 29 participants. Remarkably, 11 of the 17 were not taking medication and had sustained an average blood pressure of 122/72 mmHg, down from 145/87 mmHg. Four of the 11 unmedicated participants were medicated at baseline but did not resume medication and still maintained an average blood pressure of 114/73 mmHg. The remaining 6 people were medicated at baseline and returned to medication within the year. Moreover, the medicated group had an average blood pressure of 133/73 mmHg, which is similar to their average baseline blood pressure and higher than the average blood pressure in the unmedicated group. There were sustained improvements in body weight, body mass index (BMI), and waist circumference as well.

Given the limitations of this data, such as the small sample size and lack of control groups, it is difficult to make strong claims. Nevertheless, these results are consistent with published data[19,20] and suggest that even a single two-week water-only fasting and refeeding interven-

TABLE 6.2. **Comparison of hypertension treatments**

	SBP (mmHg)	DBP (mmHg)	SOURCE
Body weight loss*†	−3.5	−2.0	Bacon et al. (2004)[31]
Reduced alcohol intake§	−3.3	−2.0	Xin et al. (2001)[32]
Exercise†	−5.4	−3.0	Saco-Ledo et al. (2020)[33]
DASH†	−5.2	−2.6	Chiavaroli et al. (2019)[17]
Very low-calorie diet	−18	−11	Maifeld et al. (2021)[18]
Combination of low-fat, low-salt vegan diet and exercise	−17	−13	McDougall et al. (1995)[25]
Sodium restriction†	−15+	−10	Filippini et al. (2021)[34]
Combination antihypertensive medications†	−20+	−10+	Paz et al. (2016)[35]
Water-only fasting retrospective	−37	−13	Goldhamer et al. (2001)[20]
Water-only fasting prospective	−37	−10	TNHF (unpublished)[1]

Table data source: Table adopted and updated from Goldhamer et al. 2001; see reference 20. Note: DBP, diastolic blood pressure; mmHg, millimeters of mercury; SBP, systolic blood pressure.

*BP reduction per kilogram of body weight loss. †Meta-analysis. §Reduction of alcohol intake 30%–80%.

tion can result in a sustained reduction in blood pressure better than what is reported with chronic use of pharmaceutical drugs.[22] Because of these encouraging results, TNHF is conducting a first-ever, ongoing randomized controlled trial comparing the long-term effectiveness of prolonged water-only fasting to standard care (i.e., pharmaceutical drugs) in the treatment of hypertension. The ramifications could be profound: Given that SBP over 120 mmHg is associated with increased risk of death,[23] reducing high blood pressure could save thousands if not millions of lives. And although direct in-study comparisons are currently lacking, the available data indicate that prolonged water-only fasting is better at reducing blood pressure than even the most effective treatments.[13,22,24,25]

Obstacles to Establishing Fasting as an Accepted Treatment

Given the tremendous potential, it is baffling that the medical community does not actively embrace a treatment that resolves the leading cause of death as effectively as medically supervised prolonged water-only fasting. Of course, given the research limitations to date, there are reasons to be cautious. As we see it, two major obstacles have caused many clinicians and scientists to condemn the practice of prolonged water-only fasting: safety (see chapter 3) and the current medical paradigm.

Pharmaceutical companies are highly influential, and biomedical research has become dependent on the huge amounts of money spent in the hope of finding compounds and pathways that lead to the development of expensive new drugs, which can be sold as treatments and re-treatments for health problems that are expected to persist indefinitely. Conversely, prolonged water-only fasting is a holistic treatment that is relatively inexpensive and, when followed by a healthy diet and lifestyle, can resolve many health problems. From this perspective, it is plain to see that there is little financial incentive to fund or conduct prolonged water-only fasting research. Furthermore, the pharmaceutical-medical model has created a culture that expects "safety and efficacy" to be proven with double-blind, randomized (placebo) controlled trials, a.k.a. the "gold standard" of evidence.[26] However, fasting is inherently at odds with this framework because it is impossible to conduct a double-blind or placebo-controlled trial when water-only fasting is the experimental intervention; thus no amount of fasting research will ever meet this

Reductionism and Holism in Medical Practice

Reductionism is a common methodology used in research to investigate complex biological phenomena by reducing things to the sum of their individual parts. The rationale is that reducing complex systems to simpler, more "controllable" units will make them easier to comprehend. This approach, however, does not permit a thorough investigation into how complex physiological processes (which are the basis of our health) are impacted by nutrients from different combinations of foods and other factors. Medical practice has been extensively influenced by reductionist science, and people are often treated by different specialists depending on their symptoms or diagnoses.[36,37] The opposite of the reductionist approach in medical practice is a holistic approach, such as natural hygiene, which aims to understand and treat biological systems as a whole.[37]

"burden of proof." Fortunately, this is purely a methodological issue and does not mean that fasting is ineffective or even less effective than other treatments. This problem is also not unique to fasting; many alternative therapies and lifestyle changes are not considered in mainstream medicine because of methodological limitations.[27,28] The same methodological limitations would also prevent strong conclusions on the benefits of physical activity or the harms of secondhand smoking or air pollution. So, while the "gold standard" is ideal for investigating pharmaceutical drugs, it is inadequate when it comes to investigating other types of interventions.

One solution is to conduct rigorous, patient-centered research that uses randomization to compare sustained results of the entire fasting and refeeding intervention with the current standard of care rather than to a placebo control. As described earlier, this is how TNHF is researching hypertension; time will tell if the approach will be enough to successfully establish prolonged water-only fasting as a treatment for hypertension.

Conclusion

The potential for prolonged water-only fasting to treat hypertension is substantiated by compelling evidence, and we anticipate that even more robust data directly comparing fasting to the current standard of care will be forthcoming. This is no small feat given the ideological, methodological, and financial obstacles to conducting fasting research. Moreover, hypertension is just one disease! Yet even if fasting were only ever established and used as a treatment for hypertension, it would still confer tremendous benefits given the rampant and destructive nature of this disease. However, we know that fasting is a whole-body intervention that has demonstrable ability to reverse obesity and other metabolic dysfunction and offers potential in the treatment of autoimmunity and cancer as well (see chapter 7).

CASE SUMMARY

Prolonged water-only fasting enables management of severe plaque psoriasis in middle-aged man.

In addition to obesity and hypertension, prolonged water-only fasting may also improve autoimmune conditions such as psoriasis. There is no known cure for psoriasis, which is a lifelong, relapsing immune-mediated condition that causes chronic inflammation of the skin and joints. The inflammation stimulates rapid skin cell replication, leading to irritation, dryness, and formation of scales. Plaque psoriasis causes dry, itchy, scaly patches of skin. Typical treatment includes daily use of topical or oral immune-suppressing medications to prevent or prolong periods between relapses. We published a case report in the *Integrative and Complementary Therapies Journal* of a patient with a 28-year history of severe plaque psoriasis who experienced meaningful improvement in symptoms during and after a prolonged water-only fast.[29]

A 47-year-old man arrived at TrueNorth Health Center specifically to treat severe psoriasis plaques over large areas of his abdomen, right leg, right arm, and skin folds of the groin. The condition also caused painful separation of his toenail beds that bled and occasionally affected his ability to walk. These recurring symptoms were often worse during winter and times of stress. He had previously treated symptoms with topical corticosteroids, but the skin plaques and pain never resolved. Due to concerns about side effects associated with long-term steroid use, the patient discontinued use. He attempted a whole-plant-food diet, daily exercise, and a generally healthy lifestyle but experienced only minimal improvement of symptoms.

Upon arrival, his weight, BMI, and blood pressure were all within normal range, and he presented no contraindications to water-only fasting. The patient fasted for 13 days, followed by supervised refeeding on

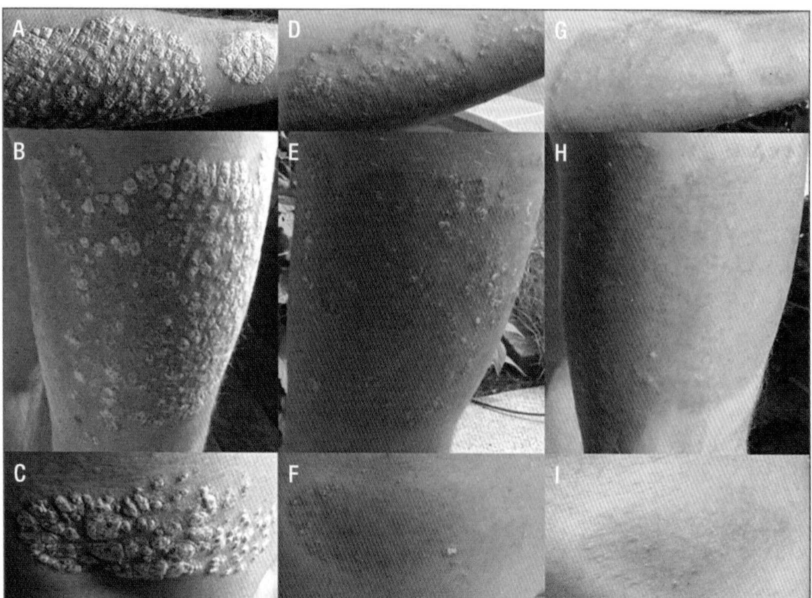

FIGURE 6.2. Psoriatic lesions on right upper forearm (A, D, G), right upper thigh (B, E, H), and upper right abdomen (C, F, I) before treatment, after treatment, and at two-month follow-up visit, respectively.

an exclusively whole-plant-food diet free of added salt, oil, and sugar (SOS-free diet) for 6 days. On the 8th day of fasting, he experienced transient stomach pain and discomfort, and he consumed vegetable and fruit juices and vegetable broth for a day before resuming the water-only fast. During the fast and throughout refeeding, the lesions improved significantly, with a decrease in scales and signs of skin renewal. He also reported improvement in arthritis and nail bed pain. At his two-month follow-up visit, the patient reported adherence to an SOS-free diet and persistent improvement of psoriatic lesions with no new developments (see figure 6.2). He also reported that this was the longest full resolution of skin plaques he had ever experienced.

The degree that fasting, diet, or their combination contributed to sustained remission of severe plaque psoriasis symptoms in this patient is unknown. Nonetheless, the results are encouraging and underscore the potential of prolonged water-only fasting and diet as an alternative treatment option for chronic psoriasis.

CHAPTER

7

The Therapeutic Potential of Fasting

Prolonged water-only fasting is an ancient practice with therapeutic potential to help us not only resolve our contemporary health crises but also gain a deeper understanding of the human body's innate physiology and capacity to heal itself. Indeed, compelling evidence from animal models—and some preliminary data in humans—indicates that fasting influences many physiological processes and phenomena, such as autophagy, apoptosis, epigenetic expression, mitochondrial function, hormone expression, immune cell function, neurogenesis, liver regeneration, and more.[1-3] In this chapter, we will explore some of these topics and how they might contribute to positive health outcomes in autoimmunity and cancer. Note that this discussion is largely theoretical, and more clinical research is needed to understand how these mechanisms impact our health.

Fortunately, we do not need to understand everything about the body's ability to heal itself in order to reap clinical benefits now. What we do need is more patient-centered research to better understand how pre-fast health status and diet, fast length and frequency, and post-fast diet influence individual outcomes. In this chapter, we will discuss how this type of research may lead to individualized treatment that will advance the clinical use of prolonged water-only fasting for health restoration. We will also discuss the use of fasting in healthy people to prevent disease in the first place. It is our hope that other scientists, clinicians, and donors gain interest in fasting and join our efforts to conduct this cutting-edge research.

Research into how prolonged water-only fasting affects our basic physiology (e.g., fat metabolism) has already uncovered some remarkably complex processes (e.g., brain ketosis).[1] It is exciting to think that additional research may lead to even more discoveries and insight into our innately intelligent response to fasting. For example, Pouneh K. Fazeli, MD, and colleagues recently found that by the 10th day of fasting, human volunteers exhibited signs of acute systemic inflammation as well as an increased number of macrophages (i.e., specialized cells that help remove pathogens and debris as well as activate innate immunity) within subcutaneous adipose tissue (other tissues were not tested).[4-6] Dr. Fazeli and colleagues also used newer technologies (e.g., RNA sequencing) to reexamine fasting metabolism and identified a decrease in the expression of genes that stimulate lipolysis under normal conditions—suggesting that fasting may shift the normal lipolytic pathway.[5]

An increase in systemic inflammation and decrease in lipolysis during the fasting process may seem paradoxical, even undesirable, when examined solely through the lens of our physiological understanding of these processes during normal conditions. However, these researchers suggest that this acute inflammatory response may reveal a helpful adaptation that activates an alternate lipolytic pathway and facilitates removal of toxic cellular debris in fat cells that is left over from the increased fat catabolism experienced during fasting. These adaptations may also contribute to beneficial health outcomes. For example, if this alternative form of lipolysis continues after food reintroduction, it may explain why all people—whether normal weight, overweight, or obese—continue losing fat while regaining lean mass, even after the fasting-refeeding interval.[7] Unfortunately, data were not collected during the post-fast refeeding period in these studies,[5] and the mechanisms responsible for continued fat loss are still unknown.

Advantageous systemic inflammation and specialized fat metabolism are just two of the fasting research topics that are ripe for exploration. We are incrementally gaining insights into these potentially significant and influential mechanisms, and research in other mammals indicates that many of these mechanisms do affect health outcomes. Currently, we don't have a solid understanding of how fasting might restore health in humans. But we do have some basic knowledge of how fasting affects other mammals and some early evidence that it helps humans too (e.g., the case summaries throughout this book). Fasting seems to improve an array of health outcomes through the interplay of numerous physiological processes, many of which begin with metabolic changes (see chapter 4). It is our intention that the discoveries described in the following section will inspire many future studies.

Does Fasting Affect Autoimmunity and Cancer through the Same Mechanisms?

Similar to strenuous physical activity, prolonged water-only fasting stresses the body, which increases transient measures of inflammation but results in a long-term reduction of inflammatory markers below starting levels.[8] For example, within 10 days of fasting, there is an increase in pro-inflammatory markers including high-sensitivity C-reactive protein (hsCRP) and cytokines that mediate systemic inflammation, including TNF-alpha, IL-10, and IL-6.[5,8,9] Not all markers have been tested beyond the end of fasting, but hsCRP decreased below starting values within 5 days of supervised refeeding and remained below pre-fast levels for at least six weeks after the intervention.[8]

Acute inflammation is part of the innate immune response to infection, trauma, and cellular abnormalities. Therefore, it follows that the acute inflammatory response initiated by fasting may start to repair damaged tissue caused by chronic inflammation. Fasting-induced inflammation may also help rebalance the immune system.[10-12] This is relevant because when the balance (i.e., number and function) of different types of immune cells is abnormal, immune tolerance, or the immune system's ability to respond appropriately to a given stimulus or environment, is compromised. In the case of autoimmunity, dysfunctional regulatory immune cells are unable to maintain control of the body's natural, self-reactive immune cell population. Effector immune cells then become intolerant and attack healthy tissue, as if it were foreign or abnormal. The reason we need a self-reactive immune system in the first place is to stop abnormal cell growth that can lead to cancer or other disorders. In the case of cancer, the immune system is too tolerant of cellular abnormalities, and growth goes unchecked. Autoimmunity and cancer also have genetic and epigenetic components that can be affected by environmental toxins, viral infections, harmful gut microbiota, or other disturbances, making treatment difficult. The concept of immune tolerance has led scientists to describe autoimmunity and cancer as two sides of the same coin; that is, they are different but related. Accordingly, there is interest in treating autoimmunity by enhancing immune tolerance to stop self-attack and treating cancer by dampening immune tolerance to start self-attack by targeting, for example, specific immune checkpoints.

Indeed, nutrient status and metabolism are closely linked to immune system function. There is also evidence that different types of fasting

What about the Microbiome?

Just as fasting has gained popularity in recent years, so has interest in the microbiome. The gut microbiome is the community of organisms found inside the gut lining of the large intestine. Many people think this solely equates to bacteria, but it includes other organisms such as yeast and viruses as well.

Recent studies have shown that our gut microbiome exists in a dynamic relationship with our body. Microbiota release metabolic byproducts, including short-chain fatty acids and other chemicals, into our digestive system, which reportedly impact human digestion, immune function, mental health, and even the aging process. But the gut microbiome is not easy to study, largely due to its diverse, dynamic, and perpetually evolving nature. Furthermore, each person maintains a relatively unique microbiome, which may respond differently, even to the same intervention. There has been a lot of microbiome research—and there is plenty more to come—but for now much of the underlying science remains unclear.[26]

Nevertheless, research has indicated that diet can affect the composition of the gut microbiome—these organisms use the food we eat for metabolic function and survival, just like we do.[27] Fasting may also impact our gut microbiome in similar ways that it impacts our cells: by affecting energy metabolism and activating processes such as autophagy. It may be that fasting allows microorganisms that thrive when we eat noxious substances (e.g., processed foods) to die off when they are no longer fed, after which a healthier biome can repopulate. Considering these possibilities, combined with potential improvements to gut wall permeability and immune function, it seems likely that fasting may benefit the gut microbiome. We are curious to find out what future research will uncover about how fasting affects the microbiome.

are able to remodel immune cell populations and modulate immune responses, perhaps by initiating the stress response and promoting self-renewal and regeneration upon food reintroduction.[12,13] Therefore, it may be that fasting and refeeding with a health-promoting diet reverses some autoimmune diseases and cancers by rebalancing the immune response, tempering activity in people with autoimmunity and elevating activity in people with certain forms of cancer. More rigorous and systematic investigations are needed to confirm this possibility, but, regardless of the mechanism, case reports support this potential.

One psoriasis case (see chapter 6) is an example of how a sufficiently long water-only fast may achieve sustained remission of unrelenting autoimmune symptoms—even after diet and lifestyle changes are unsuccessful.[14] Rheumatoid arthritis (RA) is another autoimmune condition that responds favorably to fasting, and there are even preliminary data demonstrating improvements in RA symptoms, such as reductions in joint pain and swelling, particularly during the fasting period.[15] After food reintroduction, results are less consistent, with sustained improvements in some people and a return in symptoms in others. The reason for this difference is unknown and could relate to dietary quality upon food reintroduction. More research is needed to determine which factors can worsen symptoms after fasting and if these factors can be mitigated.

There is also evidence that some types of cancer respond favorably to prolonged water-only fasting. The case summary appearing later in this chapter is especially noteworthy because it demonstrates the potential of water-only fasting and a diet free of salt, oil, and sugar (SOS-free diet) as an adjunctive therapy for follicular lymphoma.[16,17] In this case, the patient has remained disease-free, without any conventional cancer treatment, for nearly a decade. Since the publication of that report, there has been an increase in the number of people choosing to treat follicular lymphoma with prolonged water-only fasting at the TrueNorth Health Center (TNHC). However, similar to our observations into autoimmune diseases, some people have had a sustained reduction in the size and number of tumors, and some have not; there are too many confounding differences in the sample population to make a definitive conclusion. For example, there are differences in cancer type and prior treatment. Nevertheless, the results are encouraging enough that the TrueNorth Health Foundation (TNHF) is conducting a preliminary analysis to quantify if any changes are clinically meaningful and justify larger studies.

Additionally, the case of unspecified tumor regression (see chapter 4) is another example of how fasting could have possibly reversed abnormal cellular growth before it became malignant. In this case, the person completed a prolonged water-only fast during the intervening period between diagnosis and follow-up biopsy, and abnormal cellular growth began reversing. Undertaking a prolonged water-only fast during the intervening period may be sufficient to begin reversing abnormal cellular growth, as it did in this case. What's more, fasting may be beneficial in the very early stages of cancer when cells are abnormal but not yet identifiable with current screening methods. Determining if fasting would be effective in these cases requires accurate, validated

Autophagy and Apoptosis

Autophagy and apoptosis are other relevant mechanisms thought to be regulated by fasting. Autophagy is a dynamic process that degrades and recycles toxic, pathogenic, or unnecessary proteins, organelles, genetic material, microbes, and other matter from our cellular fluid. Autophagy functions to regulate amino acid availability and maintain cellular homeostasis and is of special interest because dysregulated autophagy is associated with many common diseases, including autoimmunity and cancer.[28] For example, autophagy is thought to play a complex role in both the death and survival of cancer cells depending on the stage, but the mechanisms are still being studied. Although autophagy cannot be accurately measured in humans because current methods are too invasive, indirect measures of autophagy, including large-scale gene and protein expression studies and in vitro and ex vivo autophagic flux experiments, indicate that fasting may increase autophagy in humans.[29] Fasting may increase autophagy because it depletes the available pool of intracellular amino acids[30] and reduces levels of protein acetylation,[30,31] both of which have been found to upregulate autophagy.[32-34] Given the complex role of autophagy in autoimmunity and cancer, increased autophagy during fasting may affect these diseases through unexpected or unknown mechanisms.

Apoptosis is a type of programmed cell death that is used to remove unneeded or abnormal cells; it is also thought to be activated by fasting.[35] For example, insulin-like growth factor 1 (IGF-1) is a growth factor that regulates apoptosis in model animals. IGF-1 decreases by 50% within 5 days of water-only fasting and increases to pre-fast levels within 10 days of refeeding.[24,25] One hypothesis is that decreased IGF-1 during fasting results in increased cell death.[31] Fasting is also thought to activate latent stem cells (for example, in the immune system), so that when food is reintroduced and IGF-1 levels increase, cell proliferation replaces the lost cells. The idea is that the cells that die are damaged, and the cells that grow are healthy, which will lead to beneficial health outcomes. Moreover, defective apoptosis is also thought to contribute to autoimmunity by lowering immune tolerance; as such it is possible that the enhanced apoptosis during fasting may contribute to improvements in autoimmunity by resetting immune tolerance. In time, research will show what is happening in humans.

biomarkers for early cancer detection, but these assays are still in their infancy. This may also be an effective use of fasting for the prevention of autoimmunity.

More research, including clinical trials conducted by TNHF, will help us understand these mechanisms and others as well. (Visit fasting.org to learn more about our ongoing research and clinical trials.)

Individualized Fasting and Refeeding Interventions

Prolonged water-only fasting produces measurable health improvements, with benefits reported within a single three- to four-week fasting and refeeding period.[8,18-20] A single fast and refeed, however, can't undo decades of overconsumption and disease progression. It's more likely that customizing fasting and refeeding protocols will improve immediate and sustained health outcomes for each individual.

Current prolonged water-only fasting protocols consider medical history, vital signs, symptoms, and basic blood work when screening patients and monitoring fasting progression and recovery.[21] This method effectively prevents serious adverse side effects. But what if we took it a step further? What if we used these or other biomarkers to determine the best fasting and refeeding program for each patient based on their demographic and health characteristics? Theoretically, type of fast and refeeding and maintenance diets could be tailored to an individual's state of health. Although it would certainly require a lot more research, identifying, characterizing, and validating the use of such biomarkers in different populations could help optimize each person's fasting experience.

For example, most obese people will not achieve a normal body weight during a three- to four-week fast, but they typically will lose 10% of their initial weight in that time.[8,20] Research suggests that this weight loss can be sustained for at least six weeks and that fat loss continues even when total weight loss stabilizes due to lean mass gains.[7] TNHF has also collected preliminary data from a small population in which nearly 75% of the people who were obese at the start of their fasting and refeeding intervention maintained or continued losing weight during the following year.[7] Although some results may be attributed to post-fast diet and lifestyle changes, this suggests that even one round of fasting may support long-term weight loss beyond the 5% threshold that is generally considered clinically meaningful.[22] Notably, of the 25% who had regained the weight they lost while fasting, no one rebounded beyond their starting weight.[7] Most participants lost a comparable percentage of total body weight while fasting. Future follow-up data may reveal the differences between people who gained, sustained, or lost weight over one year.

What if the goal is to reverse obesity and live at normal weight—and improve disease risk and other symptoms in the process? Would people be willing to dedicate the time required to completely normalize weight, develop new eating and lifestyle habits, and potentially restore health and quality of life once and for all? Such an objective may require prolonged water-only fasting twice a year for one to three years with dietary and lifestyle support in the intervening period until normal weight is reached or health conditions resolve. Although this may sound like a lot of effort, it is quite likely to improve health beyond the capacity of medications alone.

Type 2 diabetes is another example. Type 2 diabetes is difficult to treat because it is a late-stage manifestation of chronic, dysfunctional glucose and fat metabolism. Clinical experience indicates that a single fasting and refeeding interval is typically insufficient to completely reverse type 2 diabetes, but the intervention potentially could work as a long-term therapeutic approach. We already know that one three- to four-week interval of fasting-refeeding improved weight loss by at least 10% in obese people, double the 5% loss indicated to improve type 2 diabetes.[7,8,18,20] Now, imagine the benefits that could be gained over three to five years of regularly repeated fasting-refeeding intervals and support. Longitudinal research will help determine if repeated intervals of fasting-refeeding sufficiently normalize weight and glucose tolerance and if weight and glucose tolerance must be sustained with a yearly fasting and refeeding intervention.

How might we use biomarkers to individualize a fasting and refeeding intervention intended to fully rehabilitate a person with type 2 diabetes? One way is with biomarkers that provide information about metabolic flexibility. For example, while fasting, blood glucose and insulin levels markedly decrease, but these levels transiently spike during the immediate refeeding processes.[7,8,18,20] The levels stabilize within six weeks,[8] but the long-term effects (if any) of a transient increase in these biomarkers of insulin response are unknown. Nonetheless, preliminary data suggest that the spike is higher in people with even moderately impaired glucose metabolism. While we know that people with type 2 diabetes already have trouble with insulin before they attempt fasting, we don't know much about their post-fast insulin resistance. They might need an extended eating phase prior to fasting, a longer fasting period, or a special diet when they start eating again to reduce this insulin response. Getting more data is crucial to determining the best way to help people with type 2 diabetes during fasting and refeeding.

Far from a quick-fix health gimmick, prolonged water-only fasting, for appropriate patients, has the potential to restore health, reduce debility, and improve long-term quality of life. But it does have limitations: the longer chronic cardiovascular and metabolic diseases continue to progress, the more tissue and organ damage may occur, and the harder it becomes to reverse this damage. Humans have a remarkable capacity for cellular and tissue repair, but we can reach a limit beyond which rehabilitation is no longer possible. Therefore, it's important to begin prolonged water-only fasting as early in the disease process as possible—and better yet, before it starts.

Preventative Fasting in Healthy People

Even though many people believe they maintain a healthy lifestyle, it is estimated that only 12% of American adults are metabolically healthy, and rates of obesity and other chronic diseases increase with age.[23] Given the evidence that fasting benefits people with existing metabolic dysfunction, it may also help healthy people maintain metabolic function. Preventative fasting ideally should occur in the context of other supportive health practices (see chapter 9). There have been plenty of physiology studies, but there is a lack of clinical research assessing the benefits of fasting in already healthy people. Despite time and expense, TNHF is dedicated to longitudinal research in a large, healthy population.

Existing preliminary data indicate that prolonged water-only fasting reduces weight, including visceral fat, and may improve biomarkers of insulin sensitivity and liver health in healthy, normal-weight people.[7,18,19,24,25] Prolonged water-only fasting does not cause unexpected, sustained, or serious adverse events in healthy, normal-weight people. Notably, people who already adhere to an exclusively whole-plant-food diet before and after fasting experience continued fat loss and additional improvements in biomarkers for at least six weeks after the fasting-refeeding period. These results suggest that fasting may confer benefits beyond diet alone.

There are significant differences in some biomarkers between cardiometabolically healthy and unhealthy people. For example, although normotensive people have a reduction in blood pressure while fasting, it typically stays within normal range and quickly returns to their pre-fast values after refeeding.[7,18] In other words, even though reductions in blood pressure are sustained in hypertensive people, fasting does not cause normotensive people to become hypotensive. Another example is that during fasting, total cholesterol levels in the blood increase in normal-weight individuals but do not change in overweight or obese individuals.[7,8,18-20,24] Although the mechanism behind this difference is unknown, it does not appear to be harmful: after food reintroduction, total cholesterol returns to pre-fast levels in normal-weight people

FIGURE 7.1. **Fasting improves biomarkers in healthy people too**

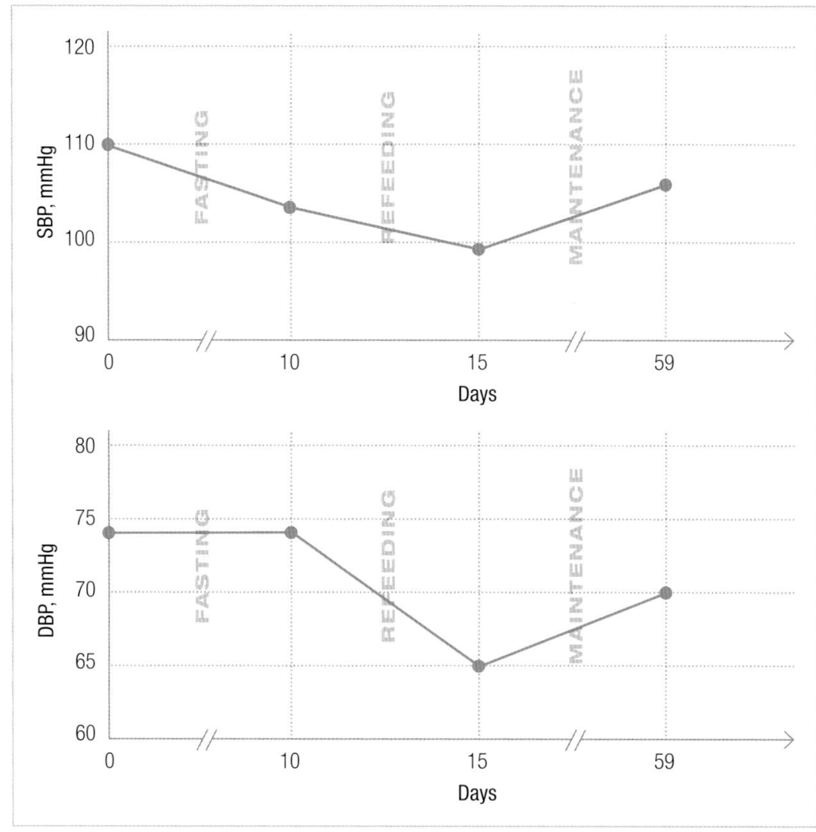

Note: Changes in systolic blood pressure (SBP), with values below 120 mmHg considered optimal, and changes in diastolic blood pressure (DBP), with values below 80 mmHg considered optimal. The average fasting, refeeding, and maintenance periods were 10, 5, and 44 days, respectively. In the maintenance period, participants were advised to follow a salt-, oil-, and sugar-free diet.[7]

and reduces significantly below pre-fast levels in overweight and obese people. These differences highlight the complex yet restorative physiological processes that take place during and after fasting, which support our health in many ways that we still do not understand.

Imagine if there were something that could help stop the crippling effects of unhealthy diet and lifestyle habits before they become serious. TNHF intends to begin a large, multiyear study to assess how repeated intervals of water-only fasting (e.g., at least five days once per year) affects the risk of developing obesity and other chronic diseases in healthy people. It is with this preventative approach that fasting may have the greatest lifesaving potential.

FIGURE 7.1. **Fasting improves biomarkers in healthy people too** (continued)

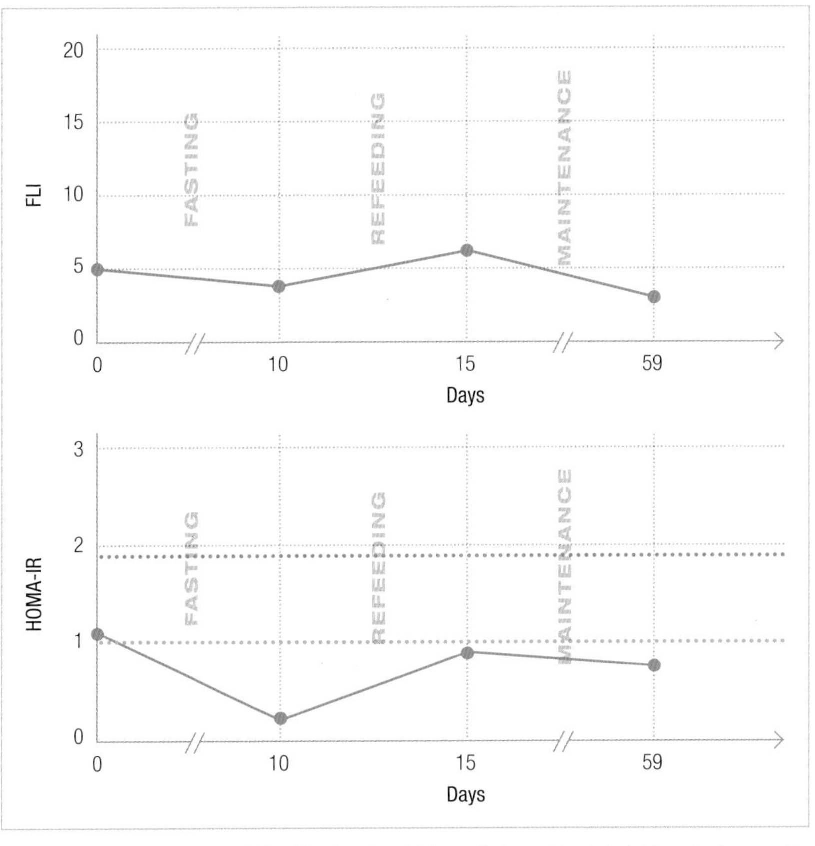

Note: Changes in fatty liver index (FLI), with values 0 to 30 (green line) considered desirable and values equal to or above 60 (not shown) denoting presence of fatty liver disease, and changes in homeostatic model assessment of insulin resistance (HOMA-IR), with values below 1.9 (red line) considered optimal insulin sensitivity. Average fasting, refeeding, and maintenance periods were 10, 5, and 44 days, respectively. In the maintenance period, participants reported eating a salt-, oil-, and sugar-free diet.[7]

Conclusion

One of the most fascinating things about prolonged water-only fasting is that it offers most humans a natural, safe way to set in motion a dynamic and progressive series of biochemical reactions that improve health. Yet there are many unanswered questions: How does the increased concentration of ketones produced during fasting affect the human brain? And how, exactly, might fasting stop and reverse tumor growth? Beyond obesity and hypertension, there are many other diseases that respond to prolonged water-only fasting but lack research. For example, there is clinical evidence that prolonged water-only fasting improves autoimmune conditions, including rheumatoid arthritis, but there is much we still do not understand about patient selection and sustaining results after the fasting period for this and other diseases. That is why TNHF will pursue the development of fasting and refeeding protocols that could improve outcomes for both healthy and unhealthy people. Although there has been more than 100 years of documented clinical study, patient-centered research remains the most important influence on the future of fasting.

CASE SUMMARY

Woman has sustained remission of stage IIIa, low-grade follicular lymphoma with prolonged water-only fasting followed by an SOS-free diet.

Follicular lymphoma (FL) is a common type of non-Hodgkin's lymphoma (NHL) that is slow growing. Most subtypes are typically incurable and follow a chronic relapse and remission pattern. Current therapies for FL, such as immunotherapy, chemotherapy, and radiation, achieve high rates of remission, but relapse rates are also high, and asymptomatic periods decrease over time. There is some evidence supporting the role of diet in the overall survival rates of FL and other cancers, but the standard of care does not include diet. We published two sequential reports in *BMJ Case Reports* of a patient with a case of low-grade FL that went into remission for at least three years following prolonged water-only fasting and an exclusively whole-plant-food, SOS-free diet.[16,17]

A 42-year-old woman arrived at TNHC five months after receiving a diagnosis of stage IIIa, low-grade FL. She was advised to do watchful waiting with observational follow-up visits every three months and sought to manage the FL with prolonged water-only fasting and diet while she waited. She did not have any contraindications and completed 21 days of water-only fasting followed by 10 days of refeeding with an SOS-free diet. By the end of the fasting and refeeding, she had lost 28 pounds (16% of her total weight) and her body mass index (BMI) decreased from 28.6 kg/m^2 to 25.3 kg/m^2. The patient was educated on and encouraged to continue following an SOS-free diet at home.

Three months later, a follow-up CT/PET scan revealed that all the previously identified lymph nodes on inguinal and axillary regions had reduced in size, and radiotracer uptake in the inguinal nodes had also decreased. The oncologist was optimistic and increased the patient's watchful waiting period to six months based on her clinical exam, blood work, and imaging. One year later, in a follow-up visit to TNHC, the patient reported that the lymph nodes remained impalpable, and she was still eating an SOS-free diet as evidenced by a continued reduction in BMI to 21.96 kg/m^2.

The second publication reported on the patient after she returned to TNHC three and a half years later and completed another prolonged water-only fast of 19 days followed by 7 days of supervised refeeding. She had not received any standard cancer treatment and remained symptom-free, with no palpable lymphadenopathy and no sign of active disease on CT/PET scans. She had also maintained her weight and continued to follow an SOS-free diet. One month after this second fast, CT/PET scans confirmed that the axillary, supraclavicular, and inguinal lymph nodes had remained normal in appearance. Plus, there was no sign of the hypermetabolic neoplasm that was seen in the scan taken two years earlier. Remarkably, when the patient returned to TNHC for a nine-year follow-up visit, she remained in remission with overall good health.

Although spontaneous regression occurs in 10% to 20% of lymphomas and cannot be ruled out, in this case the timing of the regression coincided exactly with the patient's prolonged water-only fast and significant dietary change. This case sets a precedent for considering the use of fasting and diet as a supplemental treatment in the management of FL, especially while patients are watchfully waiting, and has prompted a forthcoming case series describing positive outcomes in two additional patients.

CHAPTER 8

The Art and Science of Fasting Supervision

There are many reasons to practice or prescribe prolonged water-only fasting as a whole-body intervention: it is well tolerated, it is relatively affordable, and it improves the health of chronically ill and healthy people alike. The most common side effects are typically mild and transient, and there is very low risk of serious adverse events.[1] It is also relatively simple to implement, requiring only clean drinking water, restful accommodation, and fruits and vegetables for gradual food reintroduction. Nonetheless, medical supervision at a residential facility is the safest way to undertake a prolonged water-only fast, particularly for those who require medication weaning or management or have one or more diseases. Especially in more complicated cases, an expertly trained fasting supervisor can distinguish between common and serious side effects and symptoms.

Another reason medical supervision at a residential facility is important is that prolonged water-only fasting is a serious behavioral intervention that requires a patient to stop eating. Patients generally decide to fast after experiencing a chronic illness or the consequences of eating highly processed foods. For many, the thought of not eating may cause anxiety, especially for a first-time faster. Furthermore, eating behavior is complex, and it can be extremely difficult to control what we eat after prolonged caloric deprivation. If eating is not controlled during the refeeding process, there is a risk of electrolyte imbalance, organ failure, and refeeding syndrome, a potentially lethal condition.[2,3] Therefore, one role of the fasting supervisor is to help patients feel less anxious during their fast and stay the course during food reintroduction.

A fasting supervisor's other important role is to determine the length of the prolonged water-only fast: a patient should fast long enough to gain maximum benefit but never so long as to cause harm. A qualified fasting supervisor differentiates harmful symptoms from acute, manageable responses generated by the body in an attempt to heal itself. The supervisor also uses physical exams and lab tests to determine whether to extend, pause, or terminate the fast. Most importantly, a fasting supervisor understands the importance of not interfering with the body during the fasting process. This is a critical aspect of optimizing the fasting experience—and where the "art" of fasting supervision comes in.

Another key aspect of the art of fasting supervision is realizing that each patient is unique. It's impossible to predetermine optimal fast length or predict how an individual will respond without understanding their distinct health history. Therefore, it is imperative for the fasting supervisor to have sufficient theoretical and experiential knowledge in order to identify contraindications; select appropriate patients; safely taper and withdraw medications; correctly interpret vital signs, laboratory values, and symptoms; ensure a restful environment; prevent refeeding syndrome; and alleviate any anxiety—the patient's and their own—in order to know how to proceed with the patient's course of care. As such, the following protocol is intended solely for informational purposes and should be implemented only by practitioners with strong theoretical and experiential knowledge. Medical internship and residency training for health professionals (MD, DO, ND, DC, NP, RN, and PA) in prolonged water-only fasting supervision is available through the TrueNorth Health Foundation (TNHF). (For an outline of the full fasting protocol, see appendix 6.)

Medically Supervised Water-Only Fasting Instructions

The following is an overview of the protocol used for more than 40 years by the TrueNorth Health Center (TNHC) to ensure the safety of fasting patients.[1] In addition to eliminating caloric intake and ensuring adequate intake of drinking water, appropriate amounts of rest and controlled food reintroduction are necessary to avoid serious complications and obtain maximum benefit. Based on clinical experience as well as the results of retrospective and prospective research, this protocol has very low risk of causing a serious adverse event.[1,4] There has never been a death associated with the judicious use of this protocol and, to our knowledge, there have not been any sustained side effects.

Relative Contraindications to Fasting	
Inability to withdraw from medications	Pregnancy or nursing
Severe liver or kidney disease	Porphyria
Advanced cerebral vascular insufficiency	Higher-grade cardiac arrhythmias
Certain cancers	Active gastric ulcer disease
Medium-chain acyl-CoA dehydrogenase deficiency	Cachexia
Certain psychological disorders	Anorexia nervosa

Pre-Fast

Selecting Appropriate Patients

The best way to ensure a safe and effective fasting experience is to select appropriate patients. The ideal fasting patient is a healthy, normal-weight person who is fasting preventatively, but the unfortunate reality is that most patients are overweight or obese and chronically ill, are on multiple medications or recreational drugs, or may have toxicity from exposure to environmental or industrial chemicals. Fortunately, with proper selection, sufficient preparation, and adequate supervision, it is possible for patients with complex health conditions to safely fast.

Before a patient begins fasting, the clinician should complete a full review of their health and medical history, conduct a physical exam, and run laboratory tests, including a comprehensive metabolic panel, complete blood count, and urinalysis. This allows the clinician to rule out conditions that might contraindicate the use of fasting and provides information to help evaluate clinically important trends throughout the intervention.

Pre-Fast Diet and Medication Withdrawal

Once the patient has been properly screened and approved to fast, they should be instructed to eat only raw or steamed fruits and vegetables and to eliminate all animal products; foods with added salt, oil, and sugar; refined carbohydrates; supplements; and harmful substances such as coffee, alcohol, soda, nicotine, and other drugs for at least two days before fasting. Appropriate dietary preparation will help ease the transition to fasting and ensure that the patient is having regular bowel movements, which is important because fasting slows digestion.

The pre-fast diet can be extended for patients who are withdrawing from medications. (Often, the dietary change alone improves health enough that medication doses can be altered.) It's important to note that it is unsafe for patients to fast while taking any medications—with very few exceptions, such as thyroid medications—because the body's metabolism changes dramatically during prolonged water-only fasting. The pharmacokinetics of most drugs have not been studied in the prolonged fasting state, and the effects of drugs may be altered and cause serious complications.

Fast

Water-Only Fasting Guidelines

Once the patient has been properly prepared, medications judiciously withdrawn, and acceptable bowel and urine function established, the patient can begin the water-only fast. During this time, the patient should consume only purified water. Distilled water is preferred because it reduces the chance of contamination with microorganisms, unnecessary minerals, or toxic chemicals. The quantity of water should be dictated by thirst, but patients should drink at least 40 ounces per day to avoid dehydration. Patients who experience side effects such as nausea, emesis, or electrolyte imbalance can always consume vegetable broth free of added sodium, which is very low in calories and does not interrupt ketosis. Acaloric beverages, such as coffee and tea, should not be consumed because they are unnecessary and may negatively impact the healing process.

The patient should prioritize rest and minimize mental and physical activity. Doing activities that require a lot of energy could lead to increased loss of lean mass by increasing rates of gluconeogenesis to meet the increased need for glucose. Meditation, light stretching, and some walking are permissible and may prevent venous stasis and maintain joint and mental health. However, extreme physical activity; excessive sweating; enemas; and low-impact, high-risk activities, such as driving, are not safe. The patient may experience insomnia and should sleep whenever they are able.

Cleansing the skin with lukewarm water is permissible, but prolonged or overly hot or cold showering should be avoided to prevent orthostatic hypotension (fainting or dizziness), which can result in injuries from falls. The patient should avoid deodorants, soaps, sprays, perfumes, detergents, shampoos, toothpastes, incense, and exposure to other chemicals, which may interfere with the body's detoxification and elimination process. Patients are often more sensitive to smells and chemicals during fasting.

Bowel movements typically stop after one or two days of fasting and return a few days into food reintroduction. Enemas are not recommended, especially during fasting, in order to avoid electrolyte loss. If constipation is a concern, a longer pre-fast period of exclusively fresh fruits and vegetables should assist with elimination. Body temperature, blood pressure, and pulse and respiratory rates may drop—these are all measures of the slowing metabolic rate that occurs after several days of fasting. If needed, a hot-water bottle or heating pad can be used to help the patient stay warm.

TABLE 8.1. **Common adverse events during fasting**

MILD TO MODERATE ADVERSE EVENTS		POTENTIALLY SERIOUS ADVERSE EVENTS
A/G ratio increased	Fatigue (mild)	Abnormal electrocardiogram
Albumin increased	Headache	Delirium
ALT increased	Hematocrit increased	Diarrhea (frequent)
AST increased	Hemoglobin increased	Dyspnea due to muscle weakness
Back pain	Hypercalcemia	Fatigue (severe)
Blood bicarbonate decreased	Insomnia	Hyperkalemia (>5.5 mEq/L)
Blood bilirubin decreased	Irritability	Hypoglycemia (<45 mg/dL)
Blood bilirubin increased	Myalgia	Hypokalemia (<3 mEq/L)
BUN decreased	Nausea	Hyponatremia (<130 mEq/L)
BUN/creatinine decreased	Neutrophil count decreased	Hypotension, orthostatic
Changes in visual acuity	Palate soreness	Vomiting (frequent)
Chloride decreased	Palpitations	
Concentration impairment	Presyncope (moderate)	
Creatinine increased	Rashes	
Diarrhea	Red blood cells increased	
Dry mouth	Vomiting	
Dry skin	Water aversion	
Estimated glomerular filtration rate decreased	White blood cells decreased	

Note: A/G, albumin/globulin; ALT, alanine transaminase; AST, aspartate aminotransferase; BUN, blood urea nitrogen; mEq/L, milliequivalents per liter.

The fasting patient should be monitored for adverse signs and symptoms twice a day; body weight and vital signs, including resting blood pressure and heart rate, should be measured daily. Urinalysis, complete blood count, and comprehensive metabolic panel should be completed weekly or more frequently, as clinically indicated. Relevant symptoms should be monitored closely to prevent serious adverse events such as dehydration or low sodium. Although it is typically easy to distinguish between a common symptom and a true adverse event, this may not always be the case. Therefore, it is essential to have comprehensive knowledge of which adverse events necessitate temporarily interrupting the fast with broth or juice or require the patient to completely break the fast. If the fast has been interrupted, it can be resumed when the patient is clinically stable. This will often require a period of 48 hours or more, especially when dehydration or electrolyte issues are the complication. (For a complete list of biomarkers and how to interpret changes and respond to abnormalities during fasting, see appendix 5.)

Ideally, the patient's health status will determine the fast length. In reality, however, fast length is determined by personal factors such as willingness, finances, and time. Healthy, normal-weight patients may require only a short 5- to 10-day fast. Patients with health conditions may need to undergo several 5- to 40-day fasts with an appropriate intervening diet to obtain optimal results. Comprehensive patient education may be necessary to ensure diet and lifestyle adherence after fasting.

Post-Fast

Terminating the Water-Only Fast

Terminating a prolonged water-only fast requires the slow reintroduction of a controlled refeeding diet for a period of time equal to at least half the fast length. Proper refeeding is critical to avoid refeeding syndrome, which is associated with nutrient and electrolyte imbalances.[5,6] There is minimal research into refeeding diets, but we recommend the protocol developed at TNHC, which we have used to refeed thousands of patients (see appendix 7). This diet consists of a stepwise introduction, beginning with vegetable broths and fruit and vegetable juices, until the person is eating an exclusively whole-plant-food diet free of added salt, oil, and sugar (SOS-free diet). During gradual food reintroduction, patients should be instructed to carefully record what they eat and how they feel after eating, so that it can be reviewed by their healthcare provider. This is the perfect time to educate patients so that

Signs and Symptoms of Refeeding Syndrome	
Hypophosphatemia	Hypokalemia
Cardiac symptoms: hypotension, arrhythmias or arrest, congestive heart failure, tachycardia, EKG changes	Metabolic alkalosis
Neurological symptoms: changes in mental state, seizure, paralysis, weakness, confusion, ataxia, vertigo	Constipation, paralytic ileus
Respiratory failure	Hypomagnesemia
Muscle weakness	Gastric symptoms: abdominal pain, constipation, or diarrhea
Hematologic changes	Anemia
	Other electrolyte deficiencies
	Thiamine (vitamin B_1) deficiency
	Wernicke encephalopathy

they can establish healthy eating habits, such as eating slowly, chewing thoroughly, and limiting quantities of calorically dense foods such as nuts and seeds. Depending on their health status, some patients may begin light physical activity and gradually increase intensity.

It is normal for laboratory values to be dysregulated. For example, it is well documented that the reintroduction of food after fasting induces transient insulin resistance. These physiological changes are likely due to the metabolic switch from fat metabolism back to glucose metabolism. Therefore, it is best to wait four to six weeks before doing follow-up lab analysis to capture the most accurate assessment of the sustained clinical effects of fasting.

Conclusion

This protocol has been used to supervise fasting in more than 25,000 patients at the TNHC. Before undertaking the supervision of a fast, fasting supervisors should be well trained in pre-fast screening, tapering off medications, interpreting signs and symptoms that may arise during fasting, and reintroducing food after the fast. This will help patients achieve optimal results and avoid serious adverse events. Additionally, developing a total health-promotion program will help ensure that patients maintain benefits accrued from fasting and continue improving their health (see chapter 9).

CASE SUMMARY

An SOS-free diet as an alternative to polypharmacy for the management of chronic cardiovascular disease in an elderly man unable to fast.

In some cases, dietary change without intentional caloric restriction or fasting can result in dramatic health improvements, especially for patients who cannot fast. As we have discussed, heart disease is the most common chronic disease and the leading cause of death worldwide (see chapter 5). Current treatment guidelines include pharmaceutical therapy and lifestyle improvements. However, most physicians are inadequately trained to advise patients about lifestyle changes, and many patients, especially within the elderly population, end up taking several medications (i.e., polypharmacy) for treatment. Unfortunately, these medications fail to provide full protection against the risk of having a cardiovascular event or succumbing to premature death by any cause. Polypharmacy also contributes to the current healthcare crisis through increased medical costs, adverse drug events and interactions, medication non-adherence, decreased ability to perform activities of daily living, impaired cognition, and increased mortality.[7] Therefore, implementing lifestyle changes may improve cardiovascular disease outcomes as well as reduce the harms of polypharmacy. We published a report in *BMJ Case Reports* to this effect, describing the case of an octogenarian who normalized his biomarkers of cardiovascular health and substantially reduced medication use in fewer than six months with diet and exercise.[8] (Yes, you can still improve your health into your 80s and beyond!)

An 82-year-old man came to TNHC to improve his health and reduce the use of multiple medications. He had been diagnosed with coronary artery disease, ischemic cardiomyopathy, hyperlipidemia, hypertension, and persistent atrial fibrillation. Approximately three months before his first appointment at TNHC, he had experienced a heart attack and was treated with a stent and antiplatelet medication. After the addition of antiplatelet medication, the patient noticed a significant change in his stability, reporting that he frequently felt dizzy and lost balance. He also reported experiencing cognitive impairment, fatigue, and weakness, which diminished his quality of life. He was willing to make lifestyle changes to improve his cardiovascular health and eliminate the need for polypharmacy.

Before the patient made any dietary or lifestyle changes, he had a normal body mass index, and his blood pressure was controlled in the normal range with antihypertensive medications. He also had an irregular pulse and elevated levels of total cholesterol (TC), low-density lipoprotein (LDL), and triglycerides that remained uncontrolled despite medication use. At his initial appointment, he was advised to follow an exclusively whole-plant-food, SOS-free diet, which included unlimited raw fruits and vegetables, steamed and baked vegetables, whole grains, legumes, and small amounts of raw, unsalted nuts and seeds. He was also encouraged to get at least 30 minutes of daily physical activity. He imperfectly followed these guidelines for 12 weeks in an outpatient setting. During that time, he experienced decreases in TC and LDL, and his diuretic medication dose was halved.

Encouraged by these results, the patient decided to enroll as a resident at TNHC for nine weeks to improve adherence to the recommended diet and exercise guidelines. As an inpatient, he experienced continued improvements in hyperlipidemia and pulse rhythm. His high blood pressure also normalized without the use of antihypertensive medications. These outcomes allowed for the progressive discontinuation of statin, beta-blocker, and diuretic medications. Upon departure, he was taking only a daily dose of aspirin and an antiplatelet medication, with plans to discontinue antiplatelet treatment 12 months after the date of his heart attack, as per guidelines for acute coronary syndrome. Importantly, he reported reversal of balance issues and cognitive decline as well as symptoms associated with atrial fibrillation and ischemic cardiomyopathy, including lightheadedness, fatigue, and weakness as well as increased well-being and improved quality of life (see table 8.2).

TABLE 8.2. **Improvements in cardiovascular health and quality of life with dietary changes**

	PRETREATMENT	AFTER OUTPATIENT TREATMENT (12 WEEKS)	AFTER INPATIENT TREATMENT (9 WEEKS)
Body mass index	Normal	Normal	Normal
Blood pressure	Medicated	Medicated	Normal, unmedicated
Pulse rhythm	Irregular	Regular	Regular
Lipid panel	Abnormal	Normal	Normal
Medications	Statin Diuretic Beta-blocker Antiplatelet	Statin Diuretic (reduced) Beta-blocker Antiplatelet	Antiplatelet (with plans to discontinue)
Quality of life	Low	Medium	High

The process of deprescribing medications by introducing nonpharmaceutical medical management and gradually reducing medications is frequently dismissed as too complicated or even impossible. Although the changes reported here were not immediate, with persistence and patience and in a relatively short time, this patient was able to regain his quality of life by adhering to an SOS-free diet and increasing physical activity. This case demonstrates the potential of lifestyle change to improve markers of cardiovascular disease, allowing for the safe reduction of polypharmacy and leading to significant improvements in quality of life, particularly in the elderly.

CHAPTER

9

Optimize Your Health While Fasting and Beyond

Prolonged water-only fasting can help you establish healthy habits and break unhealthy ones. It may be the first time you will ever experience true hunger, which is an important awareness to have if you want to stop overeating. Quite likely, many of your symptoms—such as chronic pain and brain fog—will subside enough to give you a sense of what it feels like to stop overconsuming. More importantly, perhaps you will retain these benefits when you end your fast and start eating and drinking again. Gaining this experiential knowledge of your own natural intelligence can be transformative: fasting can help you reconnect with your natural state of being and support you in prioritizing long-term diet and lifestyle choices. In short, fasting on its own is beneficial, but fasting and incorporating supportive practices will help sustain your health and well-being.

Incorporating healthy practices into your daily living—before, during, and after your fast—will optimize your experience. These practices include prioritizing nutrition, hydration, sleep, physical activity, sun exposure, stress regulation, social connections, and meaningful activities. Trying to manage all these practices at once may feel overwhelming. Thankfully, the goal is not to attain perfection but to become aware, informed, and adaptable so that you can receive and interpret subtle signs from your body and make choices that support your health. You will find that this is well within your control once you develop bodily awareness and learn how to work supportive practices into your daily life. Fasting at a residential health facility, such as TrueNorth Health Center (TNHC), will give you a running start at long-term success.

In this chapter, we will review foundations of human health and our current understanding of best practices for health-promoting nutrition, hydration, sleep, movement, and sun exposure. (Stress management, connection, and meaning, which are also important, are highly dependent on the individual and more qualitative in nature; therefore, they are beyond the scope of this book.)

Nutrition

Optimal nutrition presumably results from an optimal diet. And yet an optimal diet is difficult to define because it differs from person to person, depending on their sex, age, life-cycle stage, activity level, and health status. There is certainty, however, that eating a minimally processed, whole-foods diet is absolutely critical for health.[1,2]

TNHC serves patients an exclusively whole-plant-food diet that is free of added salt, oil, and sugar (SOS-free diet). An SOS-free diet aims to provide optimal nutrition to sustain the benefits gained while water-only fasting, as well as prevent and reverse disease. An SOS-free diet is composed of 70% to 75% carbohydrates, 15% to 18% fat, and 10% to 12% protein. It is also free of processed foods, vegan or otherwise; substances such as caffeine, nicotine, and alcohol; and recreational drugs, including marijuana. Supplementation with vitamin B_{12} is necessary. An SOS-free diet promotes health by providing abundant quantities of nutrient-dense plant foods that are rich in fiber, vitamins, minerals, and phytochemicals.[3,4] Epidemiological studies and meta-analyses have identified correlations between plant-based diets and reduced risk of obesity, cardiovascular disease, type 2 diabetes, metabolic syndrome, some types of cancer, arthritis, and kidney dysfunction when compared to omnivorous diets.[5-16] Although research has not yet conclusively determined how plant-based diets prevent and reverse disease, the nutrients in plant foods are thought to improve health by lowering measures of cellular inflammation and oxidative stress and improving gut bacteria composition and metabolites.[17-20]

An SOS-free diet also eliminates added salt, oil, and sugar and limits refined carbohydrates. These substances increase the pleasurable qualities of food and contribute to a cycle of overconsumption, otherwise known as "the pleasure trap."[19] Completely removing added salt, oil, and sugar from the diet can potentially reduce the desire to overeat, especially for people who are particularly susceptible to the addictive qualities of highly processed foods. There is little doubt that diets high in sodium, sugar, and fat—especially when combined—contribute to or increase the risk of chronic degenerative diseases.[21-23] For example, high-salt diets have been shown to elevate blood pressure, decrease arte-

The Pleasure Trap

"The pleasure trap" is a term that was coined in a popular book by Drs. Doug Lisle and Alan Goldhamer to describe a cycle in which our inherent motivation to prioritize survival is hijacked by the temporary pleasure gained from harmful behaviors such as overeating highly processed foods and chronically using drugs.[19] The authors postulate that throughout human evolution, actions that increased the chance of survival—mainly food, sex, and avoidance of predation—were rewarded with short bursts of pleasurable feelings. In other words, in a natural environment, something that feels good is also good for survival. But in our contemporary environment, we have easy access to hedonic substances and behaviors that throw a wrench into this intricate machinery by stimulating reward signals in the brain. Instead of contributing to survival, however, they provide fleeting pleasure at the cost of overall health.

rial function, and impede antioxidant activity, and they are associated with increased risk of developing chronic disease.[24-27] Additionally, a recent study showed that high-salt diets negatively affect gut microbiota and immune cell function and implicates high-salt diets in exacerbating autoimmunity.[28] Studies also suggest that some types of oil consumption impair endothelial cell function, which is thought to contribute to cardiovascular disease.[29-31] Diets high in processed sugars increase biomarkers of inflammation and have been associated with increased risk of nonalcoholic fatty liver disease, cardiovascular disease, cancer, and diabetes.[32-35]

An SOS-free diet may constitute optimal nutrition, but this claim has not been substantiated. To investigate this diet, the TrueNorth Health Foundation now tracks dietary adherence in the intervening time between when research participants leave TNHC and their long-term follow-up visits. Preliminary results suggest that adherence to an SOS-free diet may have contributed to the sustained effects of prolonged water-only fasting.[36] While more research is needed, there are promising signs that an SOS-free diet is remarkably restorative.[37] (For one example, see the case summary on page 109.)

Hydration

Most people know that our bodies are made mostly of water and that staying hydrated is good for us. But how, exactly, does water promote health? The short answer is that water supports nearly all bodily functions. Describing the myriad incredible benefits of adequate hydration is outside the range of this book, but here are just a few: Water enables cell signaling, maintains blood volume and the oxygen exchange in our breath, facilitates nutrient absorption in our gut, lubricates our joints, detoxifies our bodies, and regulates our senses of taste, sight, and hearing. Adequate hydration has been linked to superior athletic performance and recovery, as well as brain performance and cognition.[38] It has also been linked to weight loss, disease prevention, and even the slowing of the aging process.[39] Conversely, inadequate hydration is associated with conditions ranging from constipation to kidney disease.[38]

Hydration needs vary from person to person, but the current recommendation is 2 liters per day for women and 3 liters per day for men.[40,41] Around 1 liter of that requirement will likely come from food consumption and metabolic output. Notably, fruits and vegetables are made up of 70% to 90% water.[38] There are also simple ways to determine your individual hydration level. The first is thirst, which is an impressive mechanism in our brains that constantly measures the water levels in the blood and lets us know when we need to drink more.[42] Another is the frequency and quality of urination, including urine color. A third measure is changes in body weight, which can be especially informative after profuse sweating.[43]

During a prolonged water-only fast, clinical experience indicates that one should consume an absolute minimum of 40 ounces, or 1.2 liters, of water per day (see chapter 8). It is important to continue drinking water while fasting to avoid dehydration, but it is possible to drink too much: drinking excessive amounts of water can lead to hyponatremia, which is characterized by low blood sodium levels. While fasting, use the quiet and stillness to monitor your thirst and urination and see for yourself if these indicators adequately inform you regarding the amount of water you need. At TNHC, patients drink only distilled water to eliminate as many contaminants as possible. Whether or not a person is fasting, daily water intake needs vary depending on stature, sweat rate, health status, and ambient environment.

Sleep and Rest

Humans function within a 24-hour cycle called the circadian rhythm, which is programmed to increase wakefulness in the daytime and promote sleepiness at night. Mechanisms activated during sleep are quintessential to hormonal balance, immune function, memory formation, and much more.[44,45] Sleep deprivation has been linked to prevalent diseases, including hypertension, diabetes, mood disorders, and dementia.[46] Human sleep studies indicate that we benefit from sleeping during the night when we are naturally inclined to do so. The exact amount of sleep people need varies with age, with adolescents requiring more sleep than adults.

You can determine if you are getting enough high-quality sleep by the total amount of uninterrupted sleep you get each night, paired with how rested you feel upon awakening. There are recent developments in how we assess sleep function, and ongoing research should help better characterize the quality of our sleep.[47] There are many ways to improve sleep hygiene, such as maintaining a regular sleep time, decreasing exposure to artificial light before sleep, and sleeping in a cool, dark, quiet place. There is evidence that avoiding meals for at least one and up to six hours before bedtime may optimize sleep.[48] Based on clinical experience, TNHC recommends avoiding meals for at least three hours before bedtime, before and after fasting, to extend the overnight fasting period.

Sleep is frequently disturbed during the night while fasting, and accordingly transient insomnia has been identified as a common adverse event.[49] It is unclear if this is because people sleep more during the day or if something else occurs during fasting. While fasting, or anytime sleep is disrupted, it is important to create a restful environment and allow yourself to rest or nap whenever possible.

Physical Activity

Regular movement is essential to good health, quite possibly because humans evolved walking and running long distances to forage and hunt for food.[50] We all know that physical activity is important; the concept is so often repeated that it has become a platitude. But it is definitely not just another platitude. We know that exercise lowers blood pressure, improves glucose tolerance, and relieves depression, among many other benefits.[51] Physical activity and fasting are similar in that they both are acute stressors that activate overlapping maintenance and repair pathways and produce similar benefits to overall health.[52-57] You could even say that fasting is like exercise without the sweat.

As with fasting and nutrition, the ideal mode, frequency, duration, and intensity of physical activity depends on each person's needs, goals, and abilities. Nonetheless, there is consensus that consistently performing various functional movements (e.g., stretching, strength building, and cardiovascular conditioning) with a burst of moderate- to vigorous-intensity movement several times each week may be the way to maximize health benefits.[55,57] *After* fasting and refeeding and throughout life, it is important to get adequate amounts of a diverse physical activity. But *during* prolonged water-only fasting, only very low-intensity physical activity is recommended. Accordingly, at TNHC patients are encouraged to engage in gentle stretching while sitting or lying down to avoid orthostatic hypotension and take slow, short walks during the day to promote healthy circulation and decrease stress.

Sunlight

Despite recommendations to use sunscreen and otherwise avoid the sun to prevent wrinkles and avoid skin cancer, getting regular sun exposure is important for our health. For example, it is well known that sun exposure is necessary for us to make vitamin D, which is a hormone involved in numerous physiological processes. Indeed, in addition to increasing vitamin D production, ultraviolet radiation elicits complex physiological responses in humans, such as regulation of the circadian rhythm and immunomodulation.[58,59] Although the research is largely inconclusive, these changes may explain some of the associations between sunlight exposure and overall state of health as underscored by observational studies that have found an association between low sun exposure and various diseases.[58] The amount of daily sun you need and the time of day you are in the sun will be largely predicated by geographical location, the seasons, and individual melanin production. But it is generally recommended to get a minimum of 15 to 30 minutes of midday sun each day or to take vitamin D_3 supplementation daily.[60] During fasting at TNHC, direct sun exposure is limited to avoid dehydration and consequent orthostatic hypotension.

Conclusion

Until very recently in evolutionary history, our environments and lifestyles were more naturally aligned with our physiology. For most people today, it is almost impossible to get adequate nutrition, hydration, sleep, exercise, sun exposure, and periods without food without an intentional effort. Prolonged water-only fasting in an environment that supports these basic practices can facilitate meeting your physiological needs over time and help you restore and maintain your health.

CASE SUMMARY

Woman improves Fuchs endothelial corneal dystrophy with an SOS-free diet.

Fuchs endothelial corneal dystrophy (FECD) is a progressive eye condition that worsens over time and may result in corneal edema, opacity, and loss of vision acuity. FECD predominantly affects women, and incidence increases with age. Treatment options are limited and aim to reduce intraocular pressure and corneal edema through medication or surgery. There are no reports of diet affecting FECD pathophysiology or improving disease outcomes. We published a case in the *International Journal of Disease Reversal and Prevention* demonstrating that long-term adherence to an exclusively whole-plant-food diet free of added salt, oil, and sugar coincided with the reversal of vision loss in a woman with FECD.

A 68-year-old woman arrived at TNHC with an 18-year history of FECD that had progressively worsened. She reported decreased visual acuity to the point of "white blindness," eye irritation, photophobia, and mild cataracts that considerably decreased her ability to complete activities of daily living. Her medical history also included obesity and hypertension. She weighed 275 pounds with a body mass index (BMI) of 46.5 kg/m^2 and her blood pressure was 143/83 mmHg. The patient was not a candidate for water-only fasting due to the inability to stop multiple medications and opted to stay at TNHC for an extended period to support strict adherence to an SOS-free diet. After only 15 days, she reported vision improvement as well as decreased itching and pain in her eyes. After she followed the diet for three months, her ophthalmologist confirmed improved visual acuity, corneal changes, decreased intraocular pressure, and resolution of edema. She continued an SOS-free diet, and her vision and other eye improvements were sustained at a follow-up visit six months later. Additionally, her weight, BMI, and blood pressure had reduced to 204 pounds, 35.2 kg/m^2, and 114/63 mmHg, respectively. This case demonstrates that dietary change alone may reverse chronic diseases that are conventionally considered unresponsive to diet and may be a potential treatment for FECD.

Conclusion

Humans can efficiently store fat when food is abundant and then metabolize that fat for energy in times of scarcity. This ability was likely the difference between life and death a million years ago, but today we habitually eat an abundance of cheap, highly processed food, pushing our metabolism and nutrient storage beyond their capacities. Consequently, humans are experiencing rates of metabolic dysfunction on a scale never before seen in history. Even though scientists are learning more about the biology of metabolic dysfunction, we do not have to understand all the details to realize that simple yet powerful habits can restore our health. These diet and lifestyle changes are effective at any stage of the health-disease continuum, but they confer their greatest value when used preventively, before chronic disease sets in.

Natural practices help restore our health because we have an innate cellular intelligence that drives biological processes as simple as repairing a paper cut and as complex as developing an adult human from a single fertilized oocyte. The best thing we can do to support these processes is to obtain physiologically appropriate amounts of nutrients, water, sleep, physical activity, and sunlight. Importantly, our bodies are also able to repair damage caused by chronic imbalance, but we must stop the behaviors that are disrupting the innate "repair" processes. Our bodies can withstand only a certain amount of damage before they can no longer fully repair themselves. This is why it is important to make changes before our particular imbalances cause irreversible harm. Luckily, our bodies are resilient and, as evidenced by the cases summarized in this book, can naturally recover even from life-altering, long-lasting conditions that mainstream medicine is often unable to treat. Fasting gives us the opportunity to reestablish equilibrium.

This truth may seem radical in a time when widespread efforts are taken to influence our food selection, medical choices, and bodily autonomy. Every day—through no fault of our own—we are inundated with dishonest marketing, fake food, toxic chemicals, and bad medical advice to the point that we have grown severely disconnected from our inherent nature. Rather than examining the underlying causes of the dysfunctions we experience, most of us—on the recommendation of trusted medical and public health professionals—throw fuel on the fire with prescription drugs and surgery. It is painfully obvious, however, that a healthcare system that thrives on prescribing pharmaceuticals to manage symptoms does not produce meaningful or sustainable health improvements: despite unprecedented medical and scientific knowledge, advanced technology, persistent medical care, and concerted drug development efforts, rates of chronic disease are historically high and continue to rise. It's baffling to think about how we ended up in a situation where what we need and what is pushed on us are so misaligned. But the truth is, managing symptoms with medication while ignoring, let alone addressing, underlying problems is highly profitable for the medical industrial complex.

Fortunately, it's possible for you to reclaim your own health. You can learn more about your body's physiological processes, listen to the "good" and "bad" signs and symptoms, and take action when these signals indicate that your body is out of balance. Try it. The next time you experience a sensation in your body that flags an imbalance, take an inventory of simple health practices (see chapter 9) and truthfully reflect on whether any changes are warranted. Then prioritize making those changes.

Obviously, making changes is easier said than done, so gaining support from family, friends, and even qualified professionals may be helpful or even necessary. In fact, that is why the TrueNorth Health Center (TNHC) was established: to provide the quiet distance from ordinary life—as well as the supervision, education, and tools—so you can hear bodily cues and take appropriate action. And whether you are decades into behaviors that have left you in terribly poor health or just want to retain the health you already have, prolonged water-only fasting, eating an SOS-free diet, and a handful of other lifestyle-related tools can help you make those changes.

It likely goes without saying, but to complete a prolonged water-only fast, you must stop eating, drinking anything but water, and drugging. Taking the time to break and modify habits is a priceless opportunity most people miss. This simple behavioral change is, in itself, powerful enough to interrupt the pleasure trap, especially for those of us trapped in poor dietary choices. The respite provided while fasting can also help people overcome their acquired distaste for natural foods and support the transition to a health-promoting diet. Indeed, many TNHC patients report that after prolonged water-only fasting, whole-plant foods taste better and dietary changes are easier to sustain.

Our research has shown that prolonged water-only fasting followed by dietary and lifestyle improvements reduced weight and blood pressure for at least six weeks and, in some cases, for at least one year following a *single* intervention. Imagine the possible outcomes if study treatment plans included repeated fasting periods and increasingly personalized interventions. Notably, the reported improvements, even with a single period of fasting, are as good as or better than what has been reported with more common interventions, such as pharmaceutical drugs. These results are incredibly encouraging, considering how poorly obesity and hypertension are currently managed. The results also begin to refute common criticisms that health improvements gained while fasting are temporary and unsustainable. Even if prolonged water-only fasting did nothing but reverse obesity and hypertension, it would still be a remarkable lifesaver, given the devastating consequences of these diseases on individuals and economies around the world.

Besides helping improve our health, fasting may actually help prevent our health from deteriorating in the first place. And although TrueNorth Health Foundation (TNHF) has preliminary data showing that water-only fasting safely reduces body fat and potentially improves biomarkers of insulin sensitivity and liver health in healthy, normal-weight people, more clinical research assessing the benefits of fasting in already healthy people is still needed.

In short, humans are not sick because we lack medical interventions. We are sick because our physiology is out of balance. We have already spent inordinate amounts of time and money trying to understand the intricacies of our pathologies, but it is more important that we understand what our physiological needs are, how to meet those needs, and ultimately, the relief and delight of feeling healthy in our bodies. Fortunately, fasting can help restore balance and reconnect us with our natural state of being. That you can stop eating for weeks and potentially avoid months or even years of debility may sound crazy. More research will reveal the degree to which this pans out, but considering that most of us have spent our entire lives overconsuming, this possibility is certainly plausible. Fasting is a medical intervention that is 100 percent natural, is relatively inexpensive, and works with your innate physiological intelligence to restore health. Prolonged water-only fasting is certainly not a panacea, but it does safely, affordably, and effectively benefit us in palpable ways.

We have personally experienced the unrivaled ability of periodic prolonged water-only fasting to improve and sustain our own health and the health of our loved ones. We hope you will consider the benefits and share this book with your medical provider, who might learn about the potentially lifesaving practice and maybe even train in the art and science of fasting supervision themselves. In the meantime, we encourage you to prioritize the natural health practices described in this book. Along with fasting, they just may save your life.

REFERENCES

CHAPTER 1

1. Fredericks R. *Fasting: An Exceptional Human Experience.* San Jose, CA: All Things Published Well, 2013.
2. Longo VD, Di Tano M, Mattson MP, Guidi N. Intermittent and periodic fasting, longevity and disease. *Nat Aging* 2021;1(1):47-59.
3. Abdelrahim DN, Rachida R, Krami AM, Nadia A, Faris ME. Sex as a biological determinant in anthropometric, biochemical, and dietary changes during Ramadan intermittent fasting in healthy people: A systematic review. *Diabetes Metab Syndr* 2023;17(5):102762.
4. Roky R, Aadil N, Krami AM, et al. Sex as a biological factor in the changes in disease patients during Ramadan intermittent fasting: A systematic review. *Front Nutr* 2022;9:908674.
5. Gupta CC, Vincent GE, Coates AM, et al. A time to rest, a time to dine: Sleep, time-restricted eating, and cardiometabolic health. *Nutrients* 2022;14(3).
6. Thomas EA, Zaman A, Sloggett KJ, et al. Early time-restricted eating compared with daily caloric restriction: A randomized trial in adults with obesity. *Obesity (Silver Spring).* 2022;30(5):1027-1038.
7. Xie Z, Sun Y, Ye Y, et al. Randomized controlled trial for time-restricted eating in healthy volunteers without obesity. *Nat Commun* 2022;13(1):1003.
8. Sun Y, Ye Y, He Y, Liu S. Time-restricted feeding: What we have done and what more we can do? *Hepatobiliary Surg Nutr* 2023;12(3):440-442.
9. Liu J, Yi P, Liu F. The effect of early time-restricted eating vs later time-restricted eating on weight loss and metabolic health. *J Clin Endocrinol Meta* 2023;108(7):1824-1834.
10. Chawla S, Beretoulis S, Deere A, Radenkovic D. The window matters: A systematic review of time restricted eating strategies in relation to cortisol and melatonin secretion. *Nutrients* 2021;13(8).
11. Cui Y, Cai T, Zhou Z, et al. Health effects of alternate-day fasting in adults: A systematic review and meta-analysis. *Front Nutr* 2020;7:586036.
12. Park J, Seo YG, Paek YJ, Song HJ, Park KH, Noh HM. Effect of alternate-day fasting on obesity and cardiometabolic risk: A systematic review and meta-analysis. *Metabolism* 2020;111:154336.
13. Patikorn C, Roubal K, Veettil SK, et al. Intermittent fasting and obesity-related health outcomes: An umbrella review of meta-analyses of randomized clinical trials. *JAMA Netw Open* 2021;4(12):e2139558.

14. Myers TR, Saul B, Karlsen M, et al. Potential effects of prolonged water-only fasting followed by a whole-plant-food diet on salty and sweet taste sensitivity and perceived intensity, food liking, and dietary intake. *Cureus* 2022;14(5):e24689.

15. Brandhorst S, Longo VD. Fasting and caloric restriction in cancer prevention and treatment. *Recent Results Cancer Res* 2016;207:241-266.

16. Longo VD, Anderson RM. Nutrition, longevity and disease: From molecular mechanisms to interventions. *Cell* 2022;185(9):1455-1470.

17. Wei M, Brandhorst S, Shelehchi M, et al. Fasting-mimicking diet and markers/risk factors for aging, diabetes, cancer, and cardiovascular disease. *Sci Transl Med* 2017;9(377).

18. Vernieri C, Fuca G, Ligorio F, et al. Fasting-mimicking diet is safe and reshapes metabolism and antitumor immunity in patients with cancer. *Cancer Discov* 2022;12(1):90-107.

19. ProLon. https://prolonfast.com/. [Accessed June 29, 2023].

20. Buchinger-Wilhelmi. Scientific documentation of Buchinger Wilhelmi therapeutic fasting. 2023. https://www.buchinger-wilhelmi.com/en/wissenschaft/.

21. Ducarmon QR, Grundler F, Le Maho Y, et al. Remodelling of the intestinal ecosystem during caloric restriction and fasting. *Trends Microbiol* 2023.

22. Grundler F, Viallon M, Mesnage R, et al. Long-term fasting: Multi-system adaptations in humans (GENESIS) study-A single-arm interventional trial. *Front Nutr* 2022;9:951000.

23. Laurens C, Grundler F, Damiot A, et al. Is muscle and protein loss relevant in long-term fasting in healthy men? A prospective trial on physiological adaptations. *J Cachexia Sarcopenia Muscle* 2021;12(6):1690-1703.

24. Grundler F, Seralini GE, Mesnage R, Peynet V, Wilhelmi de Toledo F. Excretion of heavy metals and glyphosate in urine and hair before and after long-term fasting in humans. *Front Nutr* 2021;8:708069.

25. Grundler F, Plonne D, Mesnage R, et al. Long-term fasting improves lipoprotein-associated atherogenic risk in humans. *Eur J Nutr* 2021;60(7):4031-4044.

26. Grundler F, Mesnage R, Michalsen A, Wilhelmi de Toledo F. Blood pressure changes in 1610 subjects with and without antihypertensive medication during long-term fasting. *J Am Heart Asso* 2020;9(23):e018649.

27. Grundler F, Mesnage R, Goutzourelas N, et al. Interplay between oxidative damage, the redox status, and metabolic biomarkers during long-term fasting. *Food Chem Toxicol* 2020;145:111701.

28. Wilhelmi de Toledo F, Grundler F, Goutzourelas N, et al. Influence of long-term fasting on blood redox status in humans. *Antioxidants (Basel)* 2020;9(6).

29. Mesnage R, Grundler F, Schwiertz A, Le Maho Y, Wilhelmi de Toledo F. Changes in human gut microbiota composition are linked to the energy metabolic switch during 10 d of Buchinger fasting. *J Nutr Sci* 2019;8:e36.

30. Drinda S, Grundler F, Neumann T, et al. Effects of periodic fasting on fatty liver index-A prospective observational Study. *Nutrients* 2019;11(11).

31. Viallon M, Leporq B, Drinda S, et al. Chemical-shift-encoded magnetic resonance imaging and spectroscopy to reveal immediate and long-term multi-organs composition changes of a 14-days periodic fasting intervention: A technological and case report. *Front Nutr* 2019;6:5.
32. Wilhelmi de Toledo F, Grundler F, Bergouignan A, Drinda S, Michalsen A. Safety, health improvement and well-being during a 4 to 21-day fasting period in an observational study including 1422 subjects. *PLoS One* 2019;14(1):e0209353.
33. Cahill GF, Jr. Starvation in man. *N Engl J Med* 1970;282(12):668-675.
34. Wilhelmi de Toledo F, Grundler F, Sirtori CR, Ruscica M. Unravelling the health effects of fasting: a long road from obesity treatment to healthy life span increase and improved cognition. *Ann Med* 2020;52(5):147-161.
35. Wilhelmi de Toledo F, Buchinger A, Burggrabe H, et al. Fasting therapy - an expert panel update of the 2002 consensus guidelines. *Forsch Komplementmed* 2013;20(6):434-443.
36. Steinhauser ML, Olenchock BA, O'Keefe J, et al. The circulating metabolome of human starvation. *JCI Insight* 2018;3(16).
37. Fang Y, Gu Y, Zhao C, et al. Impact of supervised beego, a traditional Chinese water-only fasting, on thrombosis and haemostasis. *BMJ Nutr Prev Health* 2021;4(1):4-17.
38. Yang C, Ma Q, Zhang H, et al. Ten days of complete fasting affected subjective sensations but not cognitive abilities in healthy adults. *Eur J Nutr* 2021;60(5):2747-2758.
39. Dai Z, Zhang H, Wu F, et al. Effects of 10-day complete fasting on physiological homeostasis, nutrition and health markers in male adults. *Nutrients* 2022;14(18).
40. Gabriel S, Ncube M, Zeiler E, et al. A six-week follow-up study on the sustained effects of prolonged water-only fasting and refeeding on markers of cardiometabolic risk. *Nutrients* 2022;14(20).
41. Letkiewicz S, Pilis K, Slezak A, et al. Eight days of water-only fasting promotes favorable changes in the functioning of the urogenital system of middle-aged healthy men. *Nutrients* 2020;13(1).
42. Mojto V, Gvozdjakova A, Kucharska J, Rausova Z, Vancova O, Valuch J. Effects of complete water fasting and regeneration diet on kidney function, oxidative stress and antioxidants. *Bratisl Lek Listy* 2018;119(2):107-111.
43. Scharf E, Zeiler E, Ncube M, et al. The effects of prolonged water-only fasting and refeeding on markers of cardiometabolic risk. *Nutrients* 2022;14(6).
44. Tang L, Li L, Bu L, et al. Bigu-style fasting affects metabolic health by modulating taurine, glucose, and cholesterol homeostasis in healthy young adults. *J Nutr* 2021;151(8):2175-2187.
45. Goldhamer A, Lisle D, Parpia B, Anderson SV, Campbell TC. Medically supervised water-only fasting in the treatment of hypertension. *J Manipulative Physiol Ther* 2001;24(5):335-339.
46. Goldhamer AC, Lisle DJ, Sultana P, et al. Medically supervised water-only fasting in the treatment of borderline hypertension. *J Altern Complement Med* 2002;8(5):643-650.

47. Finnell JS, Saul BC, Goldhamer AC, Myers TR. Is fasting safe? A chart review of adverse events during medically supervised, water-only fasting. *BMC Complement Altern Med* 2018;18(1):67.
48. Solianik R, Zidoniene K, Eimantas N, Brazaitis M. Prolonged fasting outperforms short-term fasting in terms of glucose tolerance and insulin release: a randomised controlled trial. *Br J Nutr* 2023:1-10.
49. Alexandrakis FG, Goldhamer AC, Myers TR. Challenging case in clinical practice: Water-only fasting and an exclusively whole-plant-food diet in the resolution of seborrheic keratosis. *Alt Complement Ther* 2020;26.
50. Jahrami HA, Alsibai J, Clark CCT, Faris MAE. A systematic review, meta-analysis, and meta-regression of the impact of diurnal intermittent fasting during Ramadan on body weight in healthy subjects aged 16 years and above. *Eur J Nutr* 2020;59(6):2291-2316.
51. Flanagan EW, Most J, Mey JT, Redman LM. Calorie restriction and aging in humans. *Annu Rev Nutr* 2020;40:105-133.
52. Redman LM, Ravussin E. Caloric restriction in humans: Impact on physiological, psychological, and behavioral outcomes. *Antioxid Redox Signal* 2011;14(2):275-287.

CHAPTER 2

1. Kerndt PR, Naughton JL, Driscoll CE, Loxterkamp DA. Fasting: the history, pathophysiology and complications. *West J Med* 1982;137(5):379-399.
2. Longo VD, Mattson MP. Fasting: molecular mechanisms and clinical applications. *Cell Metab* 2014;19(2):181-192.
3. Genne-Bacon EA. Thinking evolutionarily about obesity. *Yale J Biol Med* 2014;87(2):99-112.
4. Fredericks R. *Fasting: An Exceptional Human Experience.* San Jose, CA: All Things Published Well, 2013.
5. Wilson N. *Encylopedia of Ancient Greece.* New York, NY: Routledge, 2005.
6. Curran J. Review of *The Yellow Emperor's Classic of Internal Medicine. BMJ* 2008;336(7647).
7. Burfield-Hazzard L. *The Pioneers of Therapeutic Fasting in America.* Whitefish, MT: Kessinger Publishing, 2005.
8. Graham S, Trall RT, Shelton HM. *The Greatest Health Discovery.* Chicago, IL: Natural Hygiene Press, 1972.
9. Oswald JA. *Yours for Health: The Life and Times of Herbert M. Shelton.* Franklin Books, 1989.
10. Korbonits M, Blaine D, Elia M, Powell-Tuck J. Metabolic and hormonal changes during the refeeding period of prolonged fasting. *Eur J Endocrinol* 2007;157(2):157-166.
11. Nieto-Galan A. Useful charlatans: Giovanni Succi and Stefano Merlatti's fasting contest in Paris, 1886. *Sci Context* 2020;33(4):405-422.

12. Benedict FG. Chemical and physiological studies of a man fasting thirty-one days. *Proc Natl Acad Sci USA* 1915;1(4):228-231.
13. Benedict FG. A study of prolonged fasting. *Carnegie Institution of Washington Publication No 203*. 1915.
14. Bloom WL. Fasting as an introduction to the treatment of obesity. *Metabolism* 1959;8(3):214-220.
15. Stewart WK, Fleming LW. Features of a successful therapeutic fast of 382 days' duration. *Postgrad Med J* 1973;49(569):203-209.
16. Cahill GF, Jr. Fuel metabolism in starvation. *Annu Rev Nutr* 2006;26:1-22.
17. Owen OE, Morgan AP, Kemp HG, Sullivan JM, Herrera MG, Cahill GF, Jr. Brain metabolism during fasting. *J Clin Invest* 1967;46(10):1589-1595.
18. Fazeli PK, Lun M, Kim SM, et al. FGF21 and the late adaptive response to starvation in humans. *J Clin Invest* 2015;125(12):4601-4611.
19. Fazeli PK, Zhang Y, O'Keefe J, et al. Prolonged fasting drives a program of metabolic inflammation in human adipose tissue. *Mol Metab* 2020;42:101082.
20. Fazeli PK, Bredella MA, Pachon-Pena G, et al. The dynamics of human bone marrow adipose tissue in response to feeding and fasting. *JCI Insight* 2021;6(12).
21. TrueNorth Health Center. https://truenorthhealth.com. [Accessed June 29, 2023].
22. Gershfeld N, Sultana P, Goldhamer A. A case of nonpharmacologic conservative management of suspected uncomplicated subacute appendicitis in an adult male. *J Altern Complement Med* 2011;17(3):275-277.

CHAPTER 3

1. Kerndt PR, Naughton JL, Driscoll CE, et al. Fasting: the history, pathophysiology and complications. *West J Med* 1982;137(5):379-99.
2. Myers TR, Goldhamer AC. Fasting. In: MT PJM, ed. *Textbook of Natural Medicine*. 5 ed. London, England: Churchill Livingstone, 2020:293.
3. Stewart WK, Fleming LW. Features of a successful therapeutic fast of 382 days' duration. *Postgrad Med J* 1973;49(569):203-209. doi: 10.1136/pgmj.49.569.203.
4. Patikorn C, Roubal K, Veettil SK, et al. Intermittent fasting and obesity-related health outcomes: An umbrella review of meta-analyses of randomized clinical trials. *JAMA Netw Open* 2021;4(12):e2139558. doi: 10.1001/jamanetworkopen.2021.39558.
5. Flegal KM, Kit BK, Orpana H, et al. Association of all-cause mortality with overweight and obesity using standard body mass index categories: a systematic review and meta-analysis. *JAMA* 2013;309(1):71-82. doi: 10.1001/jama.2012.113905.
6. Crupi AN, Haase J, Brandhorst S, et al. Periodic and intermittent fasting in diabetes and cardiovascular disease. *Curr Diab Rep* 2020;20(12):83. doi: 10.1007/s11892-020-01362-4.

7. TrueNorth Health Center. Unpublished data.
8. Bloom WL. Fasting as an introduction to the treatment of obesity. *Metabolism* 1959;8(3):214-220.
9. Drenick EJ. Death during therapeutic starvation. *Lancet* 1968;2(7567):573. doi: 10.1016/s0140-6736(68)92438-0.
10. Hermann LS, Iversen M. Death during therapeutic starvation. *Lancet* 1968;2(7561):217. doi: 10.1016/s0140-6736(68)92649-4.
11. Spencer IO. Death during therapeutic starvation. *Lancet* 1968;2(7569): 679-680. doi: 10.1016/s0140-6736(68)92530-0.
12. Kahan A. Death during therapeutic starvation. *Lancet* 1968; letters to the editor:1378.
13. National Cancer Institute. Common Terminology Criteria for Adverse Events (CTCAE). U.S. Department of Health and Human Services, National Institutes of Health. https://ctep.cancer.gov/protocoldevelopment/electronic_applications/ctc.htm. [Accessed November 27, 2017].
14. Ezzati A, Rosenkranz SK, Phelan J, et al. The effects of isocaloric intermittent fasting vs daily caloric restriction on weight loss and metabolic risk factors for noncommunicable chronic diseases: A systematic review of randomized controlled or comparative trials. *J Acad Nutr Diet* 2023; 123(2):318-329 e1. doi: 10.1016/j.jand.2022.09.013.
15. Gudden J, Arias Vasquez A, Bloemendaal M. The effects of intermittent fasting on brain and cognitive function. *Nutrients* 2021;13(9). doi: 10.3390/nu13093166.
16. Hernon CA, Elsayed A, Vicente RM, et al. The effects of caloric restriction and/or intermittent fasting on bone health. *J Rehab Therapy* 2021;3(2):10-13.
17. Mattson MP, Longo VD, Harvie M. Impact of intermittent fasting on health and disease processes. *Ageing Res Rev* 2017;39:46-58. doi: 10.1016/j.arr.2016.10.005.
18. Park J, Seo YG, Paek YJ, et al. Effect of alternate-day fasting on obesity and cardiometabolic risk: A systematic review and meta-analysis. *Metabolism* 2020;111:154336. doi: 10.1016/j.metabol.2020.154336.
19. Dai Z, Zhang H, Wu F, et al. Effects of 10-day complete fasting on physiological homeostasis, nutrition and health markers in male adults. *Nutrients* 2022;14(18). doi: 10.3390/nu14183860.
20. Tang L, Li L, Bu L, et al. Bigu-style fasting affects metabolic health by modulating taurine, glucose, and cholesterol homeostasis in healthy young adults. *J Nutr* 2021;151(8):2175-2187. doi: 10.1093/jn/nxab123.
21. Finnell JS, Saul BC, Goldhamer AC, et al. Is fasting safe? A chart review of adverse events during medically supervised, water-only fasting. *BMC Complement Altern Med* 2018;18(1):67. doi: 10.1186/s12906-018-2136-6.
22. Jiang Y, Yang X, Dong C, et al. Five-day water-only fasting decreased metabolic-syndrome risk factors and increased anti-aging biomarkers without toxicity in a clinical trial of normal-weight individuals. *Clin Transl Med* 2021;11(8):e502. doi: 10.1002/ctm2.502.

23. Oglodek E, Pilis Prof W. Is water-only fasting safe? *Glob Adv Health Med* 2021;10:21649561211031178. doi: 10.1177/21649561211031178.

24. Ponzo V, Pellegrini M, Cioffi I, et al. The refeeding syndrome: a neglected but potentially serious condition for inpatients. A narrative review. *Intern Emerg Med* 2021;16(1):49-60. doi: 10.1007/s11739-020-02525-7.

25. Krutkyte G, Wenk L, Odermatt J, et al. Refeeding syndrome: A critical reality in patients with chronic disease. *Nutrients* 2022;14(14). doi: 10.3390/nu14142859.

26. Brazg J, Ruest A, Law S, et al. A therapeutic fast for lymphoma resulting in Wernicke encephalopathy. *J Emerg Med* 2015;49(4):471-474. doi: 10.1016/j.jemermed.2015.03.022.

27. Bhootra K, Bhootra AR, Desai K, et al. Wernicke's Encephalopathy as a part of refeeding syndrome. *J Assoc Physicians India* 2020;68(3):80-82.

28. Hutcheon DA. Malnutrition-induced Wernicke's encephalopathy following a water-only fasting diet. *Nutr Clin Pract* 2015;30(1):92-99. doi: 10.1177/0884533614561793.

29. Blanco JC, Khatri A, Kifayat A, et al. Starvation ketoacidosis due to the ketogenic diet and prolonged fasting—a possibly dangerous diet trend. *Am J Case Rep* 2019;20:1728-1731. doi: 10.12659/AJCR.917226.

30. Brett AS, Nesbit RM. A 40-day water-only fast by a Pentecostal woman: clinical and religious observations. *Am J Med Sci* 2013;345(5):418-420. doi: 10.1097/MAJ.0b013e3182760349.

31. Fazeli PK, Lun M, Kim SM, et al. FGF21 and the late adaptive response to starvation in humans. *J Clin Invest* 2015;125(12):4601-4611. doi: 10.1172/JCI83349.

32. Watanabe S, Kang DH, Feng L, et al. Uric acid, hominoid evolution, and the pathogenesis of salt-sensitivity. *Hypertension* 2002;40(3):355-360. doi: 10.1161/01.hyp.0000028589.66335.aa

33. Nery RA, Kahlow BS, Skare TL, et al. Uric acid and tissue repair. *Arq Bras Cir Dig* 2015;28(4):290-292. doi: 10.1590/S0102-6720201500040018.

34. Scharf E, Zeiler E, Ncube M, et al. The effects of prolonged water-only fasting and refeeding on markers of cardiometabolic risk. *Nutrients* 2022;14(6). doi: 10.3390/nu14061183.

35. Gabriel S, Ncube M, Zeiler E, et al. A six-week follow-up study on the sustained effects of prolonged water-only fasting and refeeding on markers of cardiometabolic risk. *Nutrients* 2022;14(20). doi: 10.3390/nu14204313.

36. Saris WH. Very-low-calorie diets and sustained weight loss. *Obes Res* 2001; 9. Suppl 4:295S-301S. doi: 10.1038/oby.2001.134.

37. El Ansari W, Elhag W. Weight regain and insufficient weight loss after bariatric surgery: Definitions, prevalence, mechanisms, predictors, prevention and management strategies, and knowledge gaps–a scoping review. *Obes Surg* 2021;31(4):1755-1766. doi: 10.1007/s11695-020-05160-5.

38. Bonjour M, Gabriel S, Goldhamer A, et al. Medically supervised, water-only fasting followed by a whole-plant-food diet reduces visceral adipose tissue. *Int J Dis Revers Prev* 2021;3(2). doi: 10.1089/107555302320825165.

39. Myers TR, Saul B, Karlsen M, et al. Potential effects of prolonged water-only fasting followed by a whole-plant-food diet on salty and sweet taste sensitivity and perceived intensity, food liking, and dietary intake. *Cureus* 2022; 14(5):e24689. doi: 10.7759/cureus.24689.

40. Korbonits M, Blaine D, Elia M, et al. Metabolic and hormonal changes during the refeeding period of prolonged fasting. *Eur J Endocrinol* 2007;157(2): 157-166. doi: 10.1530/EJE-06-0740.

41. Gajagowni S, Tarun T, Dorairajan S, et al. First report of 50-day continuous fasting in symptomatic multivessel coronary artery disease and heart failure: Cardioprotection through natural ketosis. *Mo Med* 2022;119(3):250-254.

42. Goldhamer AC, Gershfeld N, Goldman DM, et al. Challenging case in clinical practice: Long-term relief from chronic posttraumatic headache after water-only fasting and an exclusively plant-foods diet. *Alt Complement Ther* 2017;23(4).

43. National Cancer Institute. Common terminology criteria for adverse events (CTCAE). Version 5.0. U.S. Department of Health and Human Services, National Institutes of Health.

CHAPTER 4

1. Young VR, Scrimshaw NS. The physiology of starvation. *Sci Am* 1971; 225(4):14-21.

2. Lee JH, Duster M, Roberts T, et al. United States dietary trends since 1800: Lack of association between saturated fatty acid consumption and non-communicable diseases. *Front Nutr* 2021;8:748847. doi: 10.3389 /fnut.2021.748847.

3. Wu G. Amino acids: metabolism, functions, and nutrition. *Amino Acids* 2009;37(1):1-17. doi: 10.1007/s00726-009-0269-0.

4. Alves-Bezerra M, Cohen DE. Triglyceride metabolism in the liver. *Compr Physiol* 2017;8(1):1-8. doi: 10.1002/cphy.c170012.

5. Rui L. Energy metabolism in the liver. *Compr Physiol* 2014;4(1):177-197. doi: 10.1002/cphy.c130024.

6. Titchenell PM, Lazar MA, Birnbaum MJ. Unraveling the regulation of hepatic metabolism by insulin. *Trends Endocrinol Metab* 2017;28(7):497-505. doi: 10.1016/j.tem.2017.03.003.

7. Cahill GF, Jr. Fuel metabolism in starvation. *Annu Rev Nutr* 2006;26:1-22. doi: 10.1146/annurev.nutr.26.061505.111258.

8. Fazeli PK, Zhang Y, O'Keefe J, et al. Prolonged fasting drives a program of metabolic inflammation in human adipose tissue. *Mol Metab* 2020;42:101082. doi: 10.1016/j.molmet.2020.101082.

9. Fazeli PK, Bredella MA, Pachon-Pena G, et al. The dynamics of human bone marrow adipose tissue in response to feeding and fasting. *JCI Insight* 2021;6(12). doi: 10.1172/jci.insight.138636.

10. Gabriel S, Ncube M, Zeiler E, et al. A six-week follow-up study on the sustained effects of prolonged water-only fasting and refeeding on markers of cardiometabolic risk. *Nutrients* 2022;14(20). doi: 10.3390/nu14204313.

11. Bak AM, Vendelbo MH, Christensen B, et al. Prolonged fasting-induced metabolic signatures in human skeletal muscle of lean and obese men. *PLoS One* 2018;13(9):e0200817. doi: 10.1371/journal.pone.0200817.
12. Myers TR, Goldhamer AC. Fasting. In: MT PJM, ed. *Textbook of Natural Medicine*. 5 ed. London, England: Churchill Livingstone, 2020:293.
13. Owen OE, Reichard GA, Jr., Patel MS, et al. Energy metabolism in feasting and fasting. *Adv Exp Med Biol* 1979;111:169-188. doi: 10.1007/978-1-4757-0734-2_8.
14. Ahmad FB, Anderson RN. The leading causes of death in the US for 2020. *JAMA* 2021;325(18):1829-1830. doi: 10.1001/jama.2021.5469.
15. Jensen J, Rustad PI, Kolnes AJ, et al. The role of skeletal muscle glycogen breakdown for regulation of insulin sensitivity by exercise. *Front Physiol* 2011;2:112. doi: 10.3389/fphys.2011.00112.
16. Berg LC, Thomsen PD, Andersen PH, et al. Serum amyloid A is expressed in histologically normal tissues from horses and cattle. *Vet Immunol Immunopathol* 2011;144(1-2):155-159. doi: 10.1016/j.vetimm.2011.06.037.
17. Dhillon KK, Gupta S. *Biochemistry, Ketogenesis*. Treasure Island, FL: StatPearls Publishing, 2023.
18. Verdy M. Fasting in obese females. I. A study of thyroid function tests, serum proteins and electrolytes. *Can Med Assoc J* 1968;98(22):1031-1033.
19. Dai Z, Zhang H, Wu F, et al. Effects of 10-day complete fasting on physiological homeostasis, nutrition and health markers in male adults. *Nutrients* 2022;14(18). doi: 10.3390/nu14183860.
20. Pinckaers PJ, Churchward-Venne TA, Bailey D, et al. Ketone bodies and exercise performance: The next magic bullet or merely hype? *Sports Med* 2017;47(3):383-391. doi: 10.1007/s40279-016-0577-y.
21. Cahill GF, Jr. Starvation in man. *N Engl J Med* 1970;282(12):668-675. doi: 10.1056/NEJM197003192821209.
22. Varkaneh Kord H, Tinsley GM, Santos HO, et al. The influence of fasting and energy-restricted diets on leptin and adiponectin levels in humans: A systematic review and meta-analysis. *Clin Nutr* 2021;40(4):1811-1821. doi: 10.1016/j.clnu.2020.10.034.
23. Steinhauser ML, Olenchock BA, O'Keefe J, et al. The circulating metabolome of human starvation. *JCI Insight* 2018;3(16). doi: 10.1172/jci.insight.121434.
24. Fazeli PK, Faje AT, Cross EJ, et al. Serum FGF-21 levels are associated with worsened radial trabecular bone microarchitecture and decreased radial bone strength in women with anorexia nervosa. *Bone* 2015;77:6-11. doi: 10.1016/j.bone.2015.04.001.
25. Morais JBS, Dias T, Cardoso BEP, et al. Adipose tissue dysfunction: Impact on metabolic changes? *Horm Metab Res* 2022;54(12):785-794. doi: 10.1055/a-1922-7052.
26. Saltiel AR, Olefsky JM. Inflammatory mechanisms linking obesity and metabolic disease. *J Clin Invest* 2017;127(1):1-4. doi: 10.1172/JCI92035.
27. Yazici D, Sezer H. Insulin resistance, obesity and lipotoxicity. *Adv Exp Med Biol* 2017;960:277-304. doi: 10.1007/978-3-319-48382-5_12.

28. Lee YS, Olefsky J. Chronic tissue inflammation and metabolic disease. *Genes Dev* 2021;35(5-6):307-328. doi: 10.1101/gad.346312.120.

29. Martini D, Godos J, Bonaccio M, et al. Ultra-processed foods and nutritional dietary profile: A meta-analysis of nationally representative samples. *Nutrients* 2021;13(10). doi: 10.3390/nu13103390.

30. Scharf E, Zeiler E, Ncube M, et al. The effects of prolonged water-only fasting and refeeding on markers of cardiometabolic risk. *Nutrients* 2022;14(6). doi: 10.3390/nu14061183.

31. Simmons AL, Schlezinger JJ, Corkey BE. What are we putting in our food that is making us fat? Food additives, contaminants, and other putative contributors to obesity. *Curr Obes Rep* 2014;3(2):273-85. doi: 10.1007/s13679-014-0094-y.

32. Hardy OT, Czech MP, Corvera S. What causes the insulin resistance underlying obesity? *Curr Opin Endocrinol Diabetes Obes* 2012;19(2):81-87. doi: 10.1097/MED.0b013e3283514e13.

33. Leavens KF, Birnbaum MJ. Insulin signaling to hepatic lipid metabolism in health and disease. *Crit Rev Biochem Mol Biol* 2011;46(3):200-215. doi: 10.3109/10409238.2011.562481.

34. Reddy JK, Rao MS. Lipid metabolism and liver inflammation. II. Fatty liver disease and fatty acid oxidation. *Am J Physiol Gastrointest Liver Physiol* 2006;290(5):G852-G858. doi: 10.1152/ajpgi.00521.2005.

35. Samuel VT, Shulman GI. The pathogenesis of insulin resistance: Integrating signaling pathways and substrate flux. *J Clin Invest* 2016;126(1):12-22. doi: 10.1172/JCI77812.

36. Ronis MJJ, Pedersen KB, Watt J. Adverse effects of nutraceuticals and dietary supplements. *Annu Rev Pharmacol Toxicol* 2018;58:583-601. doi: 10.1146/annurev-pharmtox-010617-052844.

37. Stefanovski D, Punjabi NM, Boston RC, et al. Insulin action, glucose homeostasis and free fatty acid metabolism: Insights from a novel model. *Front Endocrinol (Lausanne)* 2021;12:625701. doi: 10.3389/fendo.2021.625701.

38. Kirk EP, Klein S. Pathogenesis and pathophysiology of the cardiometabolic syndrome. *J Clin Hypertens (Greenwich)* 2009;11(12):761-765. doi: 10.1111/j.1559-4572.2009.00054.x.

39. National Heart, Lung and Blood Institute. Metabolic Syndrome Treatment. U.S. Department of Health and Human Services, National Institutes of Health. https://www.nhlbi.nih.gov/health/metabolic-syndrome/treatment. [Updated May 27, 2022; accessed June 1, 2023].

40. Science Daily. Nearly 7 in 10 Americans Are on Prescription Drugs. June 19, 2013. Source: Mayo Clinic. https://www.sciencedaily.com/releases/2013/06/130619132352.htm.

41. Boersma P, Black LI, Ward BW. Prevalence of multiple chronic conditions among US adults, 2018. *Prev Chronic Dis* 2020;17:E106. doi: 10.5888/pcd17.200130.

42. Crosby L, Davis B, Joshi S, et al. Ketogenic diets and chronic disease: weighing the benefits against the risks. *Front Nutr* 2021;8:702802. doi: 10.3389/fnut.2021.702802.

43. Jensen NJ, Wodschow HZ, Nilsson M, et al. Effects of ketone bodies on brain metabolism and function in neurodegenerative diseases. *Int J Mol Sci* 2020;21(22). doi: 10.3390/ijms21228767.

44. Crupi AN, Haase J, Brandhorst S, et al. Periodic and intermittent fasting in diabetes and cardiovascular disease. *Curr Diab Rep* 2020;20(12):83. doi: 10.1007/s11892-020-01362-4.

45. Fang Y, Gu Y, Zhao C, et al. Impact of supervised beego, a traditional Chinese water-only fasting, on thrombosis and haemostasis. *BMJ Nutr Prev Health* 2021;4(1):4-17. doi: 10.1136/bmjnph-2020-000183.

46. Jiang Y, Yang X, Dong C, et al. Five-day water-only fasting decreased metabolic-syndrome risk factors and increased anti-aging biomarkers without toxicity in a clinical trial of normal-weight individuals. *Clin Transl Med* 2021;11(8):e502. doi: 10.1002/ctm2.502.

47. Myers TR, Butler GJ, Goldhamer A. Challenging case in clinical practice: Total resolution of hydronephrosis and ureterectasis and partial regression of an unspecified retroperitoneal mass following a medically supervised, water-only fast and an exclusively whole-plant-food diet. *Alt Complement Ther* 2020;26(1):16-18. doi: 10.1089/act.2019.29257.trm.

48. Janssen J. Hyperinsulinemia and its pivotal role in aging, obesity, type 2 diabetes, cardiovascular disease and cancer. *Int J Mol Sci* 2021;22(15). doi: 10.3390/ijms22157797.

49. Khalid M, Alkaabi J, Khan MAB, et al. Insulin signal transduction perturbations in insulin resistance. *Int J Mol Sci* 2021;22(16). doi: 10.3390/ijms 22168590.

50. Johnson AM, Olefsky JM. The origins and drivers of insulin resistance. *Cell* 2013;152(4):673-684. doi: 10.1016/j.cell.2013.01.041.

51. Freeman AM, Pennings N. *Insulin Resistance*. Treasure Island, FL: StatPearls Publishing, 2023.

52. Gayoso-Diz P, Otero-Gonzalez A, Rodriguez-Alvarez MX, et al. Insulin resistance (HOMA-IR) cut-off values and the metabolic syndrome in a general adult population: effect of gender and age: EPIRCE cross-sectional study. *BMC Endocr Disord* 2013;13:47. doi: 10.1186/1472-6823-13-47.

53. Golabi P, Paik JM, Harring M, et al. Prevalence of high and moderate risk nonalcoholic fatty liver disease among adults in the United States, 1999-2016. *Clin Gastroenterol Hepatol* 2022;20(12):2838-2847 e7. doi: 10.1016/j.cgh .2021.12.015.

54. Yu EL, Schwimmer JB. Epidemiology of pediatric nonalcoholic fatty liver disease. *Clin Liver Dis (Hoboken)* 2021;17(3):196-199. doi: 10.1002/cld.1027.

55. Cuthbertson DJ, Koskinen J, Brown E, et al. Fatty liver index predicts incident risk of prediabetes, type 2 diabetes and non-alcoholic fatty liver disease (NAFLD). *Ann Med* 2021;53(1):1256-1264. doi: 10.1080/07853890 .2021.1956685.

56. Fahed G, Aoun L, Bou Zerdan M, et al. Metabolic syndrome: Updates on pathophysiology and management in 2021. *Int J Mol Sci* 2022;23(2). doi: 10.3390/ijms23020786.

57. Hirode G, Wong RJ. Trends in the prevalence of metabolic syndrome in the United States, 2011-2016. *JAMA* 2020;323(24):2526-2528. doi: 10.1001/jama.2020.4501.
58. Ding HR, Wang JL, Ren HZ, et al. Lipometabolism and glycometabolism in liver diseases. *Biomed Res Int* 2018;2018:1287127. doi: 10.1155/2018/1287127.

CHAPTER 5

1. National Cancer Institute. Dictionary of Cancer Terms. U.S. Department of Health and Human Services, National Institutes of Health. https://www.cancer.gov/publications/dictionaries/cancer-terms/def/chronic-disease.
2. National Center for Chronic Disease Prevention and Health Promotion. Health and Economic Costs of Chronic Diseases. Centers for Disease Control and Prevention. https://www.cdc.gov/chronicdisease/about/costs/index.htm. [Accessed March 23, 2023].
3. Ahmad FB, Anderson RN. The leading causes of death in the US for 2020. *JAMA* 2021;325(18):1829-1830.
4. World Health Organization. Fact Sheet: Noncommunicable Diseases. 2022. https://www.who.int/news-room/fact-sheets/detail/noncommunicable-diseases.
5. Roser M, Ritchie H, Spooner F. Burden of disease. 2021. OurWorldInData.org. https://ourworldindata.org/burden-of-disease.
6. Hacker KA, Briss PA, Richardson L, Wright J, Petersen R. COVID-19 and chronic disease: The impact now and in the future. *Prev Chronic Dis* 2021;18:E62.
7. Reyes-Sanchez F, Basto-Abreu A, Torres-Alvarez R, et al. Fraction of COVID-19 hospitalizations and deaths attributable to chronic diseases. *Prev Med* 2022;155:106917.
8. Holman HR. The relation of the chronic disease epidemic to the health care crisis. *ACR Open Rheumatol* 2020;2(3):167-173.
9. Huebbe P, Rimbach G. Historical reflection of food processing and the role of legumes as part of a healthy balanced diet. *Foods* 2020;9(8).
10. Lee JH, Duster M, Roberts T, Devinsky O. United States dietary trends since 1800: Lack of association between saturated fatty acid consumption and non-communicable diseases. *Front Nutr* 2021;8:748847.
11. Marino M, Puppo F, Del Bo C, et al. A systematic review of worldwide consumption of ultra-processed foods: Findings and criticisms. *Nutrients* 2021;13(8).
12. Statista. Edible Oils–Worldwide. https://www.statista.com/outlook/cmo/food/oils-fats/edible-oils/worldwide#revenue. [Accessed June 28, 2023].
13. Meyers DE, Meyers BS, Chisamore TM, et al. Trends in drug revenue among major pharmaceutical companies: A 2010-2019 cohort study. *Cancer* 2022;128(2):311-316.
14. Ledley FD, McCoy SS, Vaughan G, Cleary EG. Profitability of large pharmaceutical companies compared with other large public companies. *JAMA* 2020;323(9):834-843.

15. Statista. Revenue of the Food Market Worldwide from 2014 to 2027. https://www.statista.com/forecasts/1243605/revenue-food-market-worldwide. [Accessed June 28, 2023].

16. P. P. Global Healthcare Market Research Report: Insights, Trends and Forecast 2023 – 2028. LinkedIn. February 12, 2023. https://www.linkedin.com/pulse/global-healthcare-market-research-report-insights-trends-palkhade/.

17. World Health Organization. Health Topics: Obesity. https://www.who.int/health-topics/obesity#tab=tab_1. [Accessed June 28, 2023].

18. Ellulu MS, Patimah I, Khaza'ai H, Rahmat A, Abed Y. Obesity and inflammation: The linking mechanism and the complications. *Arch Med Sci* 2017;13(4):851-863.

19. Porter SA, Massaro JM, Hoffmann U, Vasan RS, O'Donnel CJ, Fox CS. Abdominal subcutaneous adipose tissue: A protective fat depot? *Diabetes Care* 2009;32(6):1068-1075.

20. Ding C, Chan Z, Magkos F. Lean, but not healthy: The 'metabolically obese, normal-weight' phenotype. *Curr Opin Clin Nutr Metab Care* 2016;19(6):408-417.

21. Smith GI, Mittendorfer B, Klein S. Metabolically healthy obesity: Facts and fantasies. *J Clin Invest* 2019;129(10):3978-3989.

22. Woolford SJ, Sidell M, Li X, et al. Changes in body mass index among children and adolescents during the COVID-19 pandemic. *JAMA* 2021;326(14):1434-1436.

23. National Center for Health Statistics. Prevalence of Overweight, Obesity, and Severe Obesity among Adults Aged 20 and Over: United States, 1960–1962 through 2017–2018. Centers for Disease Control and Prevention. https://www.cdc.gov/nchs/data/hestat/obesity-adult-17-18/obesity-adult.htm #table1. [Accessed February 8, 2021].

24. Komlos J, Brabec M. The trend of mean BMI values of US adults, birth cohorts 1882-1986 indicates that the obesity epidemic began earlier than hitherto thought. *Am J Hum Biol* 2010;22(5):631-638.

25. Hajat C, Stein E. The global burden of multiple chronic conditions: A narrative review. *Prev Med Rep* 2018;12:284-293.

26. Knoema. Global Database on Body Mass Index (BMI). https://public.knoema.com/mqclljc/global-database-on-body-mass-index-bmi. [Accessed 2021].

27. Jaacks LM, Vandevijvere S, Pan A, et al. The obesity transition: Stages of the global epidemic. *Lancet Diabetes Endocrinol* 2019;7(3):231-240.

28. Lin X, Li H. Obesity: Epidemiology, pathophysiology, and therapeutics. *Front Endocrinol (Lausanne)* 2021;12:706978.

29. Dhurandhar NV. What is obesity? Obesity musings. *Int J Obes (Lond)* 2022;46(6):1081-1082.

30. Amato AA, Wheeler HB, Blumberg B. Obesity and endocrine-disrupting chemicals. *Endocr Connect* 2021;10(2):R87-R105.

31. Mohajer N, Du CY, Checkcinco C, Blumberg B. Obesogens: How they are identified and molecular mechanisms underlying their action. *Front Endocrinol (Lausanne)* 2021;12:780888.

32. Hall KD, Ayuketah A, Brychta R, et al. Ultra-processed diets cause excess calorie intake and weight gain: An inpatient randomized controlled trial of ad libitum food intake. *Cell Metab* 2019;30(1):67-77 e63.
33. Kladnicka I, Bludovska M, Plavinova I, Muller L, Mullerova D. Obesogens in foods. *Biomolecules* 2022;12(5).
34. Rohde K, Keller M, la Cour Poulsen L, Bluher M, Kovacs P, Bottcher Y. Genetics and epigenetics in obesity. *Metabolism* 2019;92:37-50.
35. Schwartz MW, Seeley RJ, Zeltser LM, et al. Obesity pathogenesis: An endocrine society scientific statement. *Endocr Rev* 2017;38(4):267-296.
36. Taylor R, Holman RR. Normal weight individuals who develop type 2 diabetes: The personal fat threshold. *Clin Sci (Lond)* 2015;128(7):405-410.
37. Williamson DA, Bray GA, Ryan DH. Is 5% weight loss a satisfactory criterion to define clinically significant weight loss? *Obesity (Silver Spring)* 2015; 23(12):2319-2320.
38. Shuster A, Patlas M, Pinthus JH, Mourtzakis M. The clinical importance of visceral adiposity: A critical review of methods for visceral adipose tissue analysis. *Br J Radiol* 2012;85(1009):1-10.
39. Morais JBS, Dias T, Cardoso BEP, et al. Adipose tissue dysfunction: Impact on metabolic changes? *Horm Metab Res* 2022;54(12):785-794.
40. Yazici D, Sezer H. Insulin resistance, obesity and lipotoxicity. *Adv Exp Med Biol.* 2017;960:277-304.
41. Khanna D, Khanna S, Khanna P, Kahar P, Patel BM. Obesity: A chronic low-grade inflammation and its markers. *Cureus* 2022;14(2):e22711.
42. Henein MY, Vancheri S, Longo G, Vancheri F. The role of inflammation in cardiovascular disease. *Int J Mol Sci* 2022;23(21).
43. Lee YS, Olefsky J. Chronic tissue inflammation and metabolic disease. *Genes Dev.* 2021;35(5-6):307-328.
44. Asadi A, Shadab Mehr N, Mohamadi MH, et al. Obesity and gut-microbiota-brain axis: A narrative review. *J Clin Lab Anal* 2022;36(5):e24420.
45. Martinou E, Stefanova I, Iosif E, Angelidi AM. Neurohormonal changes in the gut-brain axis and underlying neuroendocrine mechanisms following bariatric surgery. *Int J Mol Sci* 2022;23(6).
46. Haslam D. Weight management in obesity–past and present. *Int J Clin Pract* 2016;70(3):206-217.
47. De Leon A, Roemmich JN, Casperson SL. Identification of barriers to adherence to a weight loss diet in women using the nominal group technique. *Nutrients* 2020;12(12).
48. Myers TR, Saul B, Karlsen M, et al. Potential effects of prolonged water-only fasting followed by a whole-plant-food diet on salty and sweet taste sensitivity and perceived intensity, food liking, and dietary intake. *Cureus* 2022;14(5):e24689.
49. Bloom WL. Fasting as an introduction to the treatment of obesity. *Metabolism.* 1959;8(3):214-220.
50. Kerndt PR, Naughton JL, Driscoll CE, Loxterkamp DA. Fasting: The history, pathophysiology and complications. *West J Med* 1982;137(5):379-399.

51. Runcie J, Thomson TJ. Prolonged starvation—a dangerous procedure? *Br Med J* 1970;3(5720):432-435.

52. Finnell JS, Saul BC, Goldhamer AC, Myers TR. Is fasting safe? A chart review of adverse events during medically supervised, water-only fasting. *BMC Complement Altern Med* 2018;18(1):67.

53. Goldhamer AC, Gershfeld N, Goldman DM, Myers TR. Challenging case in clinical practice: Long-term relief from chronic posttraumatic headache after water-only fasting and an exclusively plant-foods diet. *Alt Complement Ther* 2017;23(4).

54. Goldhamer AC, Klaper M, Foorohar A, Myers TR. Water-only fasting and an exclusively plant foods diet in the management of stage IIIa, low-grade follicular lymphoma. *BMJ Case Rep* 2015;2015.

55. Scharf E, Zeiler E, Ncube M, et al. The effects of prolonged water-only fasting and refeeding on markers of cardiometabolic risk. *Nutrients* 2022; 14(6).

56. TrueNorth Health Foundation. Unpublished data.

57. Gabriel S, Ncube M, Zeiler E, et al. A six-week follow-up study on the sustained effects of prolonged water-only fasting and refeeding on markers of cardiometabolic risk. *Nutrients* 2022;14(20).

58. Anderson JW, Konz EC, Frederich RC, Wood CL. Long-term weight-loss maintenance: A meta-analysis of US studies. *Am J Clin Nutr* 2001;74(5): 579-584.

59. Longo VD, Di Tano M, Mattson MP, Guidi N. Intermittent and periodic fasting, longevity and disease. *Nat Aging* 2021;1(1):47-59.

60. Wilhelmi de Toledo F, Buchinger A, Burggrabe H, et al. Fasting therapy - an expert panel update of the 2002 consensus guidelines. *Forsch Komplementmed* 2013;20(6):434-443.

61. Patikorn C, Roubal K, Veettil SK, et al. Intermittent fasting and obesity-related health outcomes: An umbrella review of meta-analyses of randomized clinical trials. *JAMA Netw Open* 2021;4(12):e2139558.

62. Drew BS, Dixon AF, Dixon JB. Obesity management: Update on orlistat. *Vasc Health Risk Manag* 2007;3(6):817-821.

63. Shepherd JA, Ng BK, Sommer MJ, Heymsfield SB. Body composition by DXA. *Bone* 2017;104:101-105.

64. Tang L, Li L, Bu L, et al. Bigu-style fasting affects metabolic health by modulating taurine, glucose, and cholesterol homeostasis in healthy young adults. *J Nutr* 2021;151(8):2175-2187.

65. Bonjour M, Gabriel S, Goldhamer A, Myers TR. Medically supervised, water-only fasting followed by a whole-plant-food diet reduces visceral adipose tissue. *Int J Dis Revers Prev* 2021;3(2).

66. Collaborators GBDRF. Global, regional, and national comparative risk assessment of 84 behavioural, environmental and occupational, and metabolic risks or clusters of risks for 195 countries and territories, 1990-2017: A systematic analysis for the Global Burden of Disease Study 2017. *Lancet* 2018;392(10159):1923-1994.

67. Collaborators GBDCoD. Global, regional, and national age-sex-specific mortality for 282 causes of death in 195 countries and territories, 1980-2017: A systematic analysis for the Global Burden of Disease Study 2017. *Lancet* 2018;392(10159):1736-1788.

68. Di Rosa C, Lattanzi G, Spiezia C, et al. Mediterranean diet versus very low-calorie ketogenic diet: Effects of reaching 5% body weight loss on body composition in subjects with overweight and with obesity-a cohort study. *Int J Environ Res Public Health* 2022;19(20).

69. Centers for Disease Control and Prevention. Heart Disease Facts. 2022. https://www.cdc.gov/heartdisease/facts.htm.

70. Tsao CW, Aday AW, Almarzooq ZI, et al. Heart disease and stroke statistics-2023 update: A report from the American Heart Association. *Circulation* 2023;147(8):e93-e621.

71. International Agency for Research on Cancer. United States of America Fact Sheet. 2020. World Health Organization. https://gco.iarc.fr/today/data/factsheets/populations/840-united-states-of-america-fact-sheets.pdf.

72. American Lung Association. COPD Trends Brief: Mortality. 2020. https://www.lung.org/research/trends-in-lung-disease/copd-trends-brief/copd-mortality.

73. American Lung Association. COPD Trends Brief: Prevalence. 2020. https://www.lung.org/research/trends-in-lung-disease/copd-trends-brief/copd-prevalence.

74. Alzheimer's Association. Alzheimer's Disease Facts and Figures. https://www.alz.org/alzheimers-dementia/facts-figures. [Accessed February 16, 2024].

75. Centers for Disease Control and Prevention. National Diabetes Statistics Report. 2023. https://www.cdc.gov/diabetes/data/statistics-report/index.html.

76. Siegel RL, Miller KD, Fuchs HE, Jemal A. Cancer statistics, 2021. *CA Cancer J Clin* 2021;71(1):7-33.

77. Macrotrends. U.S. Population 1950–2023. 2023. https://www.macrotrends.net/countries/USA/united-states/population.

78. Chronic Disease Initiative. Chronic Kidney Disease in the United States. 2021. Centers for Disease Control and Prevention. https://www.cdc.gov/kidneydisease/publications-resources/ckd-national-facts.html.

79. Centers for Medicare and Medicaid Services. National Health Expenditure Data Fact Sheet. 2021. https://www.cms.gov/research-statistics-data-and-systems/statistics-trends-and-reports/nationalhealthexpenddata/nhe-fact-sheet.

80. Zippia. 25+ Incredible U.S. Pharmaceutical Statistics [2023]: Facts, Data, Trends and More. https://www.zippia.com/advice/us-pharmaceutical-statistics/. [Accessed February 21, 2023].

81. Weir CB, Jan A. *BMI Classification Percentile and Cut Off Points*. Treasure Island, FL: StatPearls Publishing, 2023.

82. World Health Organization. The SuRF Report 2: Surveillance of Chronic Disease Risk Factors. 2005. https://apps.who.int/iris/bitstream/handle/10665/43190/9241593024_eng.pdf.

CHAPTER 6

1. TrueNorth Health Foundation. Unpublished data.
2. Mills KT, Stefanescu A, He J. The global epidemiology of hypertension. *Nat Rev Nephrol* 2020;16(4):223-237. doi: 10.1038/s41581-019-0244-2.
3. Whelton SP, McEvoy JW, Shaw L, et al. Association of normal systolic blood pressure level with cardiovascular disease in the absence of risk factors. *JAMA Cardiol* 2020. doi: 10.1001/jamacardio.2020.1731.
4. Hammoud S, Kurdi M, van den Bemt BJF. Impact of fasting on cardiovascular outcomes in patients with hypertension. *J Cardiovasc Pharmacol* 2021; 78(4):481-495. doi: 10.1097/FJC.0000000000001097.
5. Ostchega Y, Fryar CD, Nwankwo T, et al. Hypertension prevalence among adults aged 18 and over: United States, 2017-2018. *NCHS Data Brief* 2020(364):1-8.
6. Huguet N, Larson A, Angier H, et al. Rates of undiagnosed hypertension and diagnosed hypertension without anti-hypertensive medication following the Affordable Care Act. *Am J Hypertens* 2021;34(9):989-998. doi: 10.1093/ajh/hpab069.
7. Chobufo MD, Gayam V, Soluny J, et al. Prevalence and control rates of hypertension in the USA: 2017-2018. *Int J Cardiol Hypertens* 2020;6:100044. doi: 10.1016/j.ijchy.2020.100044.
8. Centers for Disease Control and Prevention. Heart Disease Facts. 2022. https://www.cdc.gov/heartdisease/facts.htm.
9. Centers for Disease Control and Prevention. Health and Economic Costs of Chronic Diseases. 2023. https://www.cdc.gov/chronicdisease/about/costs/index.htm.
10. Dhakal A, Takma KC, Neupane M. Adherence to lifestyle modifications and its associated factors in hypertensive patients. *J Clin Nurs* 2022;31(15-16): 2181-2188. doi: 10.1111/jocn.16033.
11. Collaboration NCDRF. Worldwide trends in hypertension prevalence and progress in treatment and control from 1990 to 2019: A pooled analysis of 1201 population-representative studies with 104 million participants. *Lancet* 2021;398(10304):957-980. doi: 10.1016/S0140-6736(21)01330-1.
12. Ho CLB, Breslin M, Doust J, et al. Effectiveness of blood pressure-lowering drug treatment by levels of absolute risk: Post hoc analysis of the Australian National Blood Pressure Study. *BMJ Open* 2018;8(3):e017723. doi: 10.1136/bmjopen-2017-017723.
13. Bronsert MR, Henderson WG, Valuck R, et al. Comparative effectiveness of antihypertensive therapeutic classes and treatment strategies in the initiation of therapy in primary care patients: A Distributed Ambulatory Research in Therapeutics Network (DARTNet) study. *J Am Board Fam Med* 2013;26(5): 529-538. doi: 10.3122/jabfm.2013.05.130048.
14. Abegaz TM, Shehab A, Gebreyohannes EA, et al. Nonadherence to antihypertensive drugs: A systematic review and meta-analysis. *Medicine (Baltimore)* 2017;96(4):e5641. doi: 10.1097/MD.0000000000005641.

15. Albasri A, Hattle M, Koshiaris C, et al. Association between antihypertensive treatment and adverse events: Systematic review and meta-analysis. *BMJ* 2021;372(8280):n189.

16. Gebreyohannes EA, Bhagavathula AS, Abebe TB, et al. Adverse effects and non-adherence to antihypertensive medications in University of Gondar Comprehensive Specialized Hospital. *Clin Hypertens* 2019;25:1. doi: 10.1186/s40885-018-0104-6.

17. Chiavaroli L, Viguiliouk E, Nishi SK, et al. DASH dietary pattern and cardiometabolic outcomes: An umbrella review of systematic reviews and meta-analyses. *Nutrients* 2019;11(2). doi: 10.3390/nu11020338.

18. Maifeld A, Bartolomaeus H, Lober U, et al. Fasting alters the gut microbiome reducing blood pressure and body weight in metabolic syndrome patients. *Nat Commun* 2021;12(1):1970. doi: 10.1038/s41467-021-22097-0.

19. Goldhamer AC, Lisle DJ, Sultana P, et al. Medically supervised water-only fasting in the treatment of borderline hypertension. *J Altern Complement Med* 2002;8(5):643-650. doi: 10.1089/107555302320825165.

20. Goldhamer A, Lisle D, Parpia B, et al. Medically supervised water-only fasting in the treatment of hypertension. *J Manipulative Physiol Ther* 2001; 24(5):335-339. doi: 10.1067/mmt.2001.115263.

21. Finnell JS, Saul BC, Goldhamer AC, et al. Is fasting safe? A chart review of adverse events during medically supervised, water-only fasting. *BMC Complement Altern Med* 2018;18(1):67. doi: 10.1186/s12906-018-2136-6.

22. Dimmitt SB, Stampfer HG, Martin JH, et al. Efficacy and toxicity of antihypertensive pharmacotherapy relative to effective dose 50. *Br J Clin Pharmacol* 2019;85(10):2218-2227. doi: 10.1111/bcp.14033.

23. Forouzanfar MH, Liu P, Roth GA, et al. Global burden of hypertension and systolic blood pressure of at least 110 to 115 mm Hg, 1990-2015. *JAMA* 2017;317(2):165-182. doi: 10.1001/jama.2016.19043.

24. Grundler F, Mesnage R, Michalsen A, et al. Blood pressure changes in 1610 subjects with and without antihypertensive medication during long-term fasting. *J Am Heart Assoc* 2020;9(23):e018649. doi: 10.1161/JAHA.120.018649.

25. McDougall J, Litzau K, Haver E, et al. Rapid reduction of serum cholesterol and blood pressure by a twelve-day, very low fat, strictly vegetarian diet. *J Am Coll Nutr* 1995;14(5):491-496. doi: 10.1080/07315724.1995.10718541.

26. Hariton E, Locascio JJ. Randomised controlled trials—the gold standard for effectiveness research: Study design: Randomised controlled trials. *BJOG* 2018;125(13):1716. doi: 10.1111/1471-0528.15199.

27. Johnston BC, Zeraatkar D, Han MA, et al. Unprocessed red meat and processed meat consumption: Dietary guideline recommendations from the Nutritional Recommendations (NutriRECS) Consortium. *Ann Intern Med* 2019;171(10):756-764. doi: 10.7326/M19-1621.

28. Qian F, Riddle MC, Wylie-Rosett J, et al. Red and processed meats and health risks: How strong is the evidence? *Diabetes Care* 2020;43(2):265-271. doi: 10.2337/dci19-0063.

29. Bonjour M, Gabriel S, Valencia A, et al. Challenging case in clinical practice: Prolonged water-only fasting followed by an exclusively whole-plant-food diet in the management of severe plaque psoriasis. *Integr Complement Ther* 2022;28(2).

30. Whelton PK, Carey RM, Aronow WS, et al. 2017 ACC/AHA/AAPA/ABC/ACPM/AGS/APhA/ASH/ASPC/NMA/PCNA guideline for the prevention, detection, evaluation, and management of high blood pressure in adults: A report of the American College of Cardiology/American Heart Association Task Force on Clinical Practice Guidelines. *J Am Coll Cardiol* 2018;71(19): e127-e248. doi: 10.1016/j.jacc.2017.11.006.

31. Bacon SL, Sherwood A, Hinderliter A, et al. Effects of exercise, diet and weight loss on high blood pressure. *Sports Med* 2004;34(5):307-316. doi: 10.2165/00007256-200434050-00003.

32. Xin X, He J, Frontini MG, et al. Effects of alcohol reduction on blood pressure: A meta-analysis of randomized controlled trials. *Hypertension* 2001; 38(5):1112-1117. doi: 10.1161/hy1101.093424.

33. Saco-Ledo G, Valenzuela PL, Ruiz-Hurtado G, et al. Exercise reduces ambulatory blood pressure in patients with hypertension: A systematic review and meta-analysis of randomized controlled trials. *J Am Heart Assoc* 2020;9(24): e018487. doi: 10.1161/JAHA.120.018487.

34. Filippini T, Malavolti M, Whelton PK, et al. Blood pressure effects of sodium reduction: Dose-response meta-analysis of experimental studies. *Circulation* 2021;143(16):1542-1567. doi: 10.1161/CIRCULATIONAHA.120.050371.

35. Paz MA, de-La-Sierra A, Saez M, et al. Treatment efficacy of anti-hypertensive drugs in monotherapy or combination: ATOM systematic review and meta-analysis of randomized clinical trials according to PRISMA statement. *Medicine (Baltimore)* 2016;95(30):e4071. doi: 10.1097/MD.0000000000004071.

36. Fardet A, Rock E. From a reductionist to a holistic approach in preventive nutrition to define new and more ethical paradigms. *Healthcare (Basel)* 2015; 3(4):1054-1063. doi: 10.3390/healthcare3041054.

37. Ahn AC, Tewari M, Poon CS, et al. The limits of reductionism in medicine: Could systems biology offer an alternative? *PLoS Med* 2006;3(6):e208. doi: 10.1371/journal.pmed.0030208.

CHAPTER 7

1. Longo VD, Anderson RM. Nutrition, longevity and disease: From molecular mechanisms to interventions. *Cell* 2022;185(9):1455-1470. doi: 10.1016/j.cell.2022.04.002.

2. Longo VD, Cortellino S. Fasting, dietary restriction, and immunosenescence. *J Allergy Clin Immunol* 2020;146(5):1002-1004. doi: 10.1016/j.jaci.2020.07.035.

3. Longo VD, Di Tano M, Mattson MP, et al. Intermittent and periodic fasting, longevity and disease. *Nat Aging* 2021;1(1):47-59. doi: 10.1038/s43587-020-00013-3.

4. Bredella MA, Buckless C, Fazeli PK, et al. Bone marrow adipose tissue composition following high-caloric feeding and fasting. *Bone* 2021;152:116093. doi: 10.1016/j.bone.2021.116093.
5. Fazeli PK, Zhang Y, O'Keefe J, et al. Prolonged fasting drives a program of metabolic inflammation in human adipose tissue. *Mol Metab* 2020;42:101082. doi: 10.1016/j.molmet.2020.101082.
6. Zhang C, Yang M, Ericsson AC. Function of macrophages in disease: current understanding on molecular mechanisms. *Front Immunol* 2021;12:620510. doi: 10.3389/fimmu.2021.620510.
7. Zeiler E, Gabriel S, Ncube M, et al. Prolonged water-only fasting is a safe and feasible treatment option for managing stage 1 and 2 hypertension. medXriv 2024;Preprint. doi: 10.1101/2024.02.04.24302309.
8. Gabriel S, Ncube M, Zeiler E, et al. A six-week follow-up study on the sustained effects of prolonged water-only fasting and refeeding on markers of cardiometabolic risk. *Nutrients* 2022;14(20) doi: 10.3390/nu14204313.
9. Borkowska A, Tomczyk M, Zychowska M, et al. Effect of 8-day fasting on leukocytes expression of genes and proteins involved in iron metabolism in healthy men. *Int J Mol Sci* 2021;22(6) doi: 10.3390/ijms22063248.
10. Soliman AM, Barreda DR. Acute inflammation in tissue healing. *Int J Mol Sci* 2022;24(1). doi: 10.3390/ijms24010641.
11. Horwitz DA, Fahmy TM, Piccirillo CA, et al. Rebalancing immune homeostasis to treat autoimmune diseases. *Trends Immunol* 2019;40(10):888-908. doi: 10.1016/j.it.2019.08.003.
12. Buono R, Longo VD. When fasting gets tough, the tough immune cells get going-or die. *Cell* 2019;178(5):1038-1040. doi: 10.1016/j.cell.2019.07.052.
13. Okawa T, Nagai M, Hase K. Dietary intervention impacts immune cell functions and dynamics by inducing metabolic rewiring. *Front Immunol* 2020;11:623989. doi: 10.3389/fimmu.2020.623989.
14. Bonjour M, Gabriel S, Valencia A, et al. Challenging case in clinical practice: Prolonged water-only fasting followed by an exclusively whole-plant-food diet in the management of severe plaque psoriasis. *Integr Complement Ther* 2022;28(2).
15. Uden AM, Trang L, Venizelos N, et al. Neutrophil functions and clinical performance after total fasting in patients with rheumatoid arthritis. *Ann Rheum Dis* 1983;42(1):45-51. doi: 10.1136/ard.42.1.45.
16. Goldhamer AC, Klaper M, Foorohar A, et al. Water-only fasting and an exclusively plant foods diet in the management of stage IIIa, low-grade follicular lymphoma. *BMJ Case Rep* 2015;2015. doi: 10.1136/bcr-2015-211582.
17. Myers TR, Zittel M, Goldhamer AC. Follow-up of water-only fasting and an exclusively plant food diet in the management of stage IIIa, low-grade follicular lymphoma. *BMJ Case Rep* 2018;2018. doi: 10.1136/bcr-2018-225520.
18. Dai Z, Zhang H, Wu F, et al. Effects of 10-day complete fasting on physiological homeostasis, nutrition and health markers in male adults. *Nutrients* 2022;14(18). doi: 10.3390/nu14183860.

19. Fang Y, Gu Y, Zhao C, et al. Impact of supervised beego, a traditional Chinese water-only fasting, on thrombosis and haemostasis. *BMJ Nutr Prev Health* 2021;4(1):4-17. doi: 10.1136/bmjnph-2020-000183.

20. Scharf E, Zeiler E, Ncube M, et al. The effects of prolonged water-only fasting and refeeding on markers of cardiometabolic risk. *Nutrients* 2022; 14(6). doi: 10.3390/nu14061183.

21. Finnell JS, Saul BC, Goldhamer AC, et al. Is fasting safe? A chart review of adverse events during medically supervised, water-only fasting. *BMC Complement Altern Med* 2018;18(1):67. doi: 10.1186/s12906-018-2136-6.

22. Williamson DA, Bray GA, Ryan DH. Is 5% weight loss a satisfactory criterion to define clinically significant weight loss? *Obesity (Silver Spring)* 2015; 23(12):2319-2320. doi: 10.1002/oby.21358.

23. Araujo J, Cai J, Stevens J. Prevalence of optimal metabolic health in American adults: National Health and Nutrition Examination Survey 2009-2016. *Metab Syndr Relat Disord* 2019;17(1):46-52. doi: 10.1089/met.2018.0105.

24. Tang L, Li L, Bu L, et al. Bigu-style fasting affects metabolic health by modulating taurine, glucose, and cholesterol homeostasis in healthy young adults. *J Nutr* 2021;151(8):2175-2187. doi: 10.1093/jn/nxab123.

25. Jiang Y, Yang X, Dong C, et al. Five-day water-only fasting decreased metabolic-syndrome risk factors and increased anti-aging biomarkers without toxicity in a clinical trial of normal-weight individuals. *Clin Transl Med* 2021; 11(8):e502. doi: 10.1002/ctm2.502.

26. Ducarmon QR, Grundler F, Le Maho Y, et al. Remodelling of the intestinal ecosystem during caloric restriction and fasting. *Trends Microbiol* 2023; 31(8):832-844. doi: 10.1016/j.tim.2023.02.009.

27. David LA, Maurice CF, Carmody RN, et al. Diet rapidly and reproducibly alters the human gut microbiome. *Nature* 2014;505(7484):559-563. doi: 10.1038/nature12820.

28. Perrotta C, Cattaneo MG, Molteni R, et al. Autophagy in the regulation of tissue differentiation and homeostasis. *Front Cell Dev Biol* 2020;8:602901. doi: 10.3389/fcell.2020.602901.

29. Walter S, Jung T, Herpich C, et al. Determination of the autophagic flux in murine and human peripheral blood mononuclear cells. *Front Cell Dev Biol* 2023;11:1122998. doi: 10.3389/fcell.2023.1122998.

30. Giesecke K, Magnusson I, Ahlberg M, et al. Protein and amino acid metabolism during early starvation as reflected by excretion of urea and methylhistidines. *Metabolism* 1989;38(12):1196-1200. doi: 10.1016/0026-0495(89) 90159-5.

31. Pietrocola F, Demont Y, Castoldi F, et al. Metabolic effects of fasting on human and mouse blood in vivo. *Autophagy* 2017;13(3):567-578. doi: 10.1080 /15548627.2016.1271513.

32. Son SM, Park SJ, Stamatakou E, et al. Leucine regulates autophagy via acetylation of the mTORC1 component raptor. *Nat Commun* 2020;11(1):3148. doi: 10.1038/s41467-020-16886-2.

33. Son SM, Park SJ, Fernandez-Estevez M, et al. Autophagy regulation by acetylation-implications for neurodegenerative diseases. *Exp Mol Med* 2021; 53(1): 30-41. doi: 10.1038/s12276-021-00556-4.
34. Liu C, Ji L, Hu J, et al. Functional amino acids and autophagy: Diverse signal transduction and application. *Int J Mol Sci* 2021;22(21). doi: 10.3390/ijms222111427.
35. Qi J, Chen X, Wu Q, et al. Fasting induces hepatocellular carcinoma cell apoptosis by inhibiting SET8 expression. *Oxid Med Cell Longev* 2020; 2020:3985089. doi: 10.1155/2020/3985089.

CHAPTER 8

1. Finnell JS, Saul BC, Goldhamer AC, Myers TR. Is fasting safe? A chart review of adverse events during medically supervised, water-only fasting. *BMC Complement Altern Med* 2018;18(1):67.
2. Korbonits M, Blaine D, Elia M, Powell-Tuck J. Metabolic and hormonal changes during the refeeding period of prolonged fasting. *Eur J Endocrinol* 2007;157(2):157-166.
3. Bhootra K, Bhootra AR, Desai K, Bhootra RK, R MS. Wernicke's encephalopathy as a part of refeeding syndrome. *J Assoc Physicians India* 2020;68(3): 80-82.
4. TrueNorth Health Foundation. Unpublished data.
5. Krutkyte G, Wenk L, Odermatt J, Schuetz P, Stanga Z, Friedli N. Refeeding syndrome: A critical reality in patients with chronic disease. *Nutrients* 2022;14(14).
6. Ponzo V, Pellegrini M, Cioffi I, Scaglione L, Bo S. The refeeding syndrome: A neglected but potentially serious condition for inpatients. A narrative review. *Intern Emerg Med* 2021;16(1):49-60.
7. Maher RL, Hanlon J, Hajjar ER. Clinical consequences of polypharmacy in elderly. *Expert Opin Drug Saf* 2014;13(1):57-65.
8. Beauchesne AB, Goldhamer AC, Myers TR. Exclusively plant, whole-food diet for polypharmacy due to persistent atrial fibrillation, ischaemic cardiomyopathy, hyperlipidaemia and hypertension in an octogenarian. *BMJ Case Rep* 2018;11(1).

CHAPTER 9

1. U.S. Department of Health and Human Services. Dietary Guidelines for Americans, 2020-2025. 9th Edition. December 2020. https://www.dietaryguidelines.gov/resources/2020-2025-dietary-guidelines-online-materials.
2. World Health Organization. Healthy Diet. 2020. https://www.who.int/news-room/fact-sheets/detail/healthy-diet.
3. Minich DM. A review of the science of colorful, plant-based food and practical strategies for "eating the rainbow." *J Nutr Metab* 2019;2019:2125070.

4. Schwingshackl L, Schwedhelm C, Hoffmann G, et al. Food groups and risk of all-cause mortality: A systematic review and meta-analysis of prospective studies. *Am J Clin Nutr* 2017;105(6):1462-1473.
5. Benatar JR, Stewart RAH. Cardiometabolic risk factors in vegans; a meta-analysis of observational studies. *PLoS One* 2018;13(12):e0209086.
6. Chen X, Wei G, Jalili T, et al. The associations of plant protein intake with all-cause mortality in CKD. *Am J Kidney Dis* 2016;67(3):423-430.
7. Chiavaroli L, Nishi SK, Khan TA, et al. Portfolio dietary pattern and cardiovascular disease: A systematic review and meta-analysis of controlled trials. *Prog Cardiovasc Dis* 2018;61(1):43-53.
8. Clinton CM, O'Brien S, Law J, Renier CM, Wendt MR. Whole-foods, plant-based diet alleviates the symptoms of osteoarthritis. *Arthritis* 2015; 2015:708152.
9. Dinu M, Abbate R, Gensini GF, Casini A, Sofi F. Vegetarian, vegan diets and multiple health outcomes: A systematic review with meta-analysis of observational studies. *Crit Rev Food Sci Nutr* 2017;57(17):3640-3649.
10. Esselstyn CB, Jr., Gendy G, Doyle J, Golubic M, Roizen MF. A way to reverse CAD? *J Fam Pract* 2014;63(7):356-364b.
11. Fraser GE. Vegetarian diets: What do we know of their effects on common chronic diseases? *Am J Clin Nutr* 2009;89(5):1607S-1612S.
12. Le LT, Sabate J. Beyond meatless, the health effects of vegan diets: Findings from the Adventist cohorts. *Nutrients* 2014;6(6):2131-2147.
13. McEvoy CT, Temple N, Woodside JV. Vegetarian diets, low-meat diets and health: A review. *Public Health Nutr* 2012;15(12):2287-2294.
14. Ornish D, Scherwitz LW, Billings JH, et al. Intensive lifestyle changes for reversal of coronary heart disease. *JAMA.* 1998;280(23):2001-2007.
15. Philippou E, Nikiphorou E. Are we really what we eat? Nutrition and its role in the onset of rheumatoid arthritis. *Autoimmun Rev.* 2018;17(11):1074-1077.
16. Sofi F, Dinu M, Pagliai G, et al. Low-calorie vegetarian versus Mediterranean diets for reducing body weight and improving cardiovascular risk profile: CARDIVEG Study (Cardiovascular Prevention With Vegetarian Diet). *Circulation.* 2018;137(11):1103-1113.
17. Benzie IF, Wachtel-Galor S. Vegetarian diets and public health: Biomarker and redox connections. *Antioxid Redox Signal* 2010;13(10):1575-1591.
18. Eichelmann F, Schwingshackl L, Fedirko V, Aleksandrova K. Effect of plant-based diets on obesity-related inflammatory profiles: A systematic review and meta-analysis of intervention trials. *Obes Rev.* 2016;17(11):1067-1079.
19. Lisle DJ, Goldhamer A. *The Pleasure Trap.* Summertown, TN: Healthy Living Publications, 2006.
20. Tomova A, Bukovsky I, Rembert E, et al. The effects of vegetarian and vegan diets on gut microbiota. *Front Nutr.* 2019;6:47.
21. Chiuve SE, Fung TT, Rimm EB, et al. Alternative dietary indices both strongly predict risk of chronic disease. *J Nutr.* 2012;142(6):1009-1018.

22. Collaborators GBDD. Health effects of dietary risks in 195 countries, 1990-2017: A systematic analysis for the Global Burden of Disease Study 2017. *Lancet* 2019;393(10184):1958-1972.

23. Schulze MB, Martinez-Gonzalez MA, Fung TT, Lichtenstein AH, Forouhi NG. Food based dietary patterns and chronic disease prevention. *BMJ*. 2018; 361:k2396.

24. Delahaye F. Should we eat less salt? *Arch Cardiovasc Dis*. 2013;106(5): 324-332.

25. Derkach A, Sampson J, Joseph J, Playdon MC, Stolzenberg-Solomon RZ. Effects of dietary sodium on metabolites: The Dietary Approaches to Stop Hypertension (DASH)-Sodium Feeding Study. *Am J Clin Nutr.* 2017;106(4): 1131-1141.

26. DuPont JJ, Greaney JL, Wenner MM, et al. High dietary sodium intake impairs endothelium-dependent dilation in healthy salt-resistant humans. *J Hypertens*. 2013;31(3):530-536.

27. Robinson AT, Edwards DG, Farquhar WB. The influence of dietary salt beyond blood pressure. *Curr Hypertens Rep*. 2019;21(6):42.

28. Wilck N, Matus MG, Kearney SM, et al. Salt-responsive gut commensal modulates T(H)17 axis and disease. *Nature*. 2017;551(7682):585-589.

29. Chen KL, Jung P, Kulkoyluoglu-Cotul E, et al. Impact of diet and nutrition on cancer hallmarks. *J Cancer Prev Curr Res*. 2017;7(4).

30. Nagao M, Asai A, Sugihara H, Oikawa S. Fat intake and the development of type 2 diabetes. *Endocr J* 2015;62(7):561-572.

31. Wu JHY, Micha R, Mozaffarian D. Dietary fats and cardiometabolic disease: Mechanisms and effects on risk factors and outcomes. *Nat Rev Cardiol* 2019; 16(10):581-601.

32. Abid A, Taha O, Nseir W, Farah R, Grosovski M, Assy N. Soft drink consumption is associated with fatty liver disease independent of metabolic syndrome. *J Hepatol* 2009;51(5):918-924.

33. Basu S, Yoffe P, Hills N, Lustig RH. The relationship of sugar to population-level diabetes prevalence: An econometric analysis of repeated cross-sectional data. *PLoS One* 2013;8(2):e57873.

34. Howard BV, Wylie-Rosett J. Sugar and cardiovascular disease: A statement for healthcare professionals from the Committee on Nutrition of the Council on Nutrition, Physical Activity, and Metabolism of the American Heart Association. *Circulation* 2002;106(4):523-527.

35. Yang Q, Zhang Z, Gregg EW, Flanders WD, Merritt R, Hu FB. Added sugar intake and cardiovascular diseases mortality among US adults. *JAMA Intern Med* 2014;174(4):516-524.

36. Gabriel S, Ncube M, Zeiler E, et al. A six-week follow-up study on the sustained effects of prolonged water-only fasting and refeeding on markers of cardiometabolic risk. *Nutrients*. 2022;14(20).

37. Myers TR, Beauchesne AB, Goldhamer A. An exclusively whole-plant-food diet in the improvement of Fuchs' endothelial corneal dystrophy. *International Journal of Disease Reversal and Prevention* 2020;2(1):4.

38. Popkin BM, D'Anci KE, Rosenberg IH. Water, hydration, and health. *Nutr Rev* 2010;68(8):439-458.

39. Dmitrieva NI, Gagarin A, Liu D, Wu CO, Boehm M. Middle-age high normal serum sodium as a risk factor for accelerated biological aging, chronic diseases, and premature mortality. *EBioMedicine* 2023;87:104404.

40. Authority EFS. Scientific opinion on dietary reference values for water. *EFSA Journal* 2010;8(3):1459.

41. Medicine Io. *Dietary Reference Intakes for Water, Potassium, Sodium, Chloride, and Sulfate* Washington, DC: The National Academies Press, 2005.

42. Zimmerman CA, Leib DE, Knight ZA. Neural circuits underlying thirst and fluid homeostasis. *Nat Rev Neurosci* 2017;18(8):459-469.

43. Armstrong LE. Hydration assessment techniques. *Nutr Rev* 2005;63(6 Pt 2): S40-S54.

44. Longo VD, Panda S. Fasting, circadian rhythms, and time-restricted feeding in healthy lifespan. *Cell Metab* 2016;23(6):1048-1059.

45. Rasch B, Born J. About sleep's role in memory. *Physiol Rev* 2013;93(2): 681-766.

46. Grandner MA. Sleep, health, and society. *Sleep Med Clin* 2020;15(2): 319-340.

47. Snyder E, Cai B, DeMuro C, Morrison MF, Ball W. A new single-item sleep quality scale: Results of psychometric evaluation in patients with chronic primary insomnia and depression. *J Clin Sleep Med* 2018;14(11):1849-1857.

48. Iao SI, Jansen E, Shedden K, et al. Associations between bedtime eating or drinking, sleep duration and wake after sleep onset: Findings from the American time use survey. *Br J Nutr* 2021;127(12):1-10.

49. Finnell JS, Saul BC, Goldhamer AC, Myers TR. Is fasting safe? A chart review of adverse events during medically supervised, water-only fasting. *BMC Complement Altern Med* 2018;18(1):67.

50. Bramble DM, Lieberman DE. Endurance running and the evolution of Homo. *Nature* 2004;432(7015):345-352.

51. Booth FW, Roberts CK, Laye MJ. Lack of exercise is a major cause of chronic diseases. *Compr Physiol* 2012;2(2):1143-1211.

52. Peake JM, Markworth JF, Nosaka K, Raastad T, Wadley GD, Coffey VG. Modulating exercise-induced hormesis: Does less equal more? *J Appl Physiol (1985)* 2015;119(3):172-189.

53. Powers SK, Jackson MJ. Exercise-induced oxidative stress: Cellular mechanisms and impact on muscle force production. *Physiol Rev* 2008;88(4):1243-1276.

54. Paffenbarger RS, Jr., Hyde RT, Wing AL, Hsieh CC. Physical activity, all-cause mortality, and longevity of college alumni. *N Engl J Med.* 1986;314(10): 605-613.

55. Piercy KL, Troiano RP, Ballard RM, et al. The Physical Activity Guidelines for Americans. *JAMA.* 2018;320(19):2020-2028.

56. Sheng M, Yang J, Bao M, et al. The relationships between step count and all-cause mortality and cardiovascular events: A dose-response meta-analysis. *J Sport Health Sci.* 2021;10(6):620-628.

57. Garber CE, Blissmer B, Deschenes MR, et al. American College of Sports Medicine position stand. Quantity and quality of exercise for developing and maintaining cardiorespiratory, musculoskeletal, and neuromotor fitness in apparently healthy adults: guidance for prescribing exercise. *Med Sci Sports Exerc.* 2011;43(7):1334-1359.

58. Hart PH, Norval M, Byrne SN, Rhodes LE. Exposure to ultraviolet radiation in the modulation of human diseases. *Annu Rev Pathol* 2019;14:55-81.

59. Nikkola V, Miettinen ME, Karisola P, et al. Ultraviolet B radiation modifies circadian time in epidermal skin and in subcutaneous adipose tissue. *Photodermatol Photoimmunol Photomed* 2019;35(3):157-163.

60. National Institutes of Health. Vitamin D. 2023. https://ods.od.nih.gov/factsheets/VitaminD-HealthProfessional/.

GLOSSARY

abstinence The practice of self-restraint.

acute disease A disease process that is rapid, sudden, and short in duration (e.g., bone fracture or asthma attack).

adherence The degree to which a patient follows medical directives or advice, such as proper medication use.

adipokines A group of signaling molecules, hormones, or cytokines, secreted by fat cells (adipocytes) that can have pro- or anti-inflammatory properties and play a role in regulating satiety, fat distribution, and insulin sensitivity, among others.

adiponectin A type of adipokine (or type of hormone secreted by fat cells) involved in regulation of glucose and fatty acid metabolism and known to have anti-inflammatory properties.

adverse advent An unfavorable symptom or laboratory finding that emerges or occurs during the use of a medical treatment (e.g., pharmaceutical drugs) or procedure (e.g., surgery). Adverse event reporting during clinical trials can help assess the safety of an intervention.

allopathic Another term for *conventional medicine*, *modern medicine*, or *Western medicine*.

alpha-ketoacids Acids made from amino acids structured in the alpha configuration, they are precursor molecules in the TCA (or Krebs) cycle. These are different molecules, made from different precursors than ketones.

alternate-day fasting (ADF) A type of intermittent fast that alternates between one fast day and one feast day.

amino acids Smaller molecules that are the building blocks of proteins. There are 20 amino acids, 9 of which are essential and come from the diet. All proteins are made by some combination of these 20 amino acids.

anabolic reaction A chemical reaction in which smaller or simpler molecules are combined to create larger structural or storage molecules. This process uses energy.

autoimmune A condition in which the body's immune system attacks healthy tissue or cells by mistake. This process leads to inflammation.

autophagy A biological process that removes or recycles unwanted cellular material while preserving cellular structure.

biomarker A measurable molecule within the body that can be used as an indicator or predictor of health conditions or disease.

caloric restriction A process by which daily caloric intake is kept below what is typically recommended while still maintaining needed daily nutrients.

case report A scientific report detailing a new or unusual circumstance, such as a sign, symptom, diagnosis, or treatment of one patient.

catabolic reaction A chemical reaction whereby larger molecules are broken down into smaller molecules. This process releases energy.

chronic disease A disease process that has a long duration, typically persisting for more than three months.

chylomicron A type of lipoprotein that is produced by enterocytes and transports dietary fat molecules.

circadian rhythm Biological changes that occur within a 24-hour cycle.

communicable disease A transmissible or infectious disease that "spreads" from person to person, animal to person, and so on.

cytokine Molecules that are secreted and play a role in cell-to-cell signaling (a.k.a. cellular signaling).

de novo Latin, "from new." The process of making a molecule that usually is obtained from the diet "from scratch" using molecules found within the cell.

ectopic Occurring outside its normal location.

endocrine Glands that secrete hormones.

endogenous In biology, something that originates from inside the body.

enterocytes Cell types that line the intestinal wall.

enzyme Protein molecules that facilitate or accelerate a chemical reaction.

epidemiological study The study of patterns or behaviors on health or disease of a given population.

epigenetic Modifications of genetic material (e.g., DNA) that respond to environmental changes.

exogenous In biology, something that originates from outside the body.

fast (noun) The partial or total cessation of caloric intake.

fasting-mimicking diet (FMD) A type of diet designed to mimic a prolonged fast by increasing ketone levels without completely eliminating caloric intake.

fatty acid hydrolysis A chemical reaction during which larger fat molecules (triglycerides) are broken down into smaller fat particles (fatty acids), which can later be used to produce adenosine triphosphate (ATP) or energy.

fatty acid oxidation (beta-oxidation) A chemical reaction during which an electron is lost is referred to as oxidation. Beta-oxidation is a catabolic reaction occurring within the mitochondria of the cell, where fatty acid molecules are broken down for energy.

gluconeogenesis A chemical reaction that uses noncarbohydrate molecules to create new glucose molecules that can be used to generate adenosine triphosphate (ATP) through glycolysis. The noncarbohydrate sources are generated from fat and protein catabolism.

glycerol A carbon-containing chemical compound that is part of sugar alcohols. This is the building block for lipids.

glycogen A type of storage molecule comprised of many "branches" of glucose; in humans, glycogen is stored in liver or muscle cells.

glycogenesis *Genesis* means "to create." Glycogenesis is a set of chemical reactions that combine many glucose molecules to form glycogen, a larger molecule used for glucose storage.

glycogenolysis *Lysis* means "to break down." Glycogenolysis is a set of chemical reactions that break down glycogen into smaller molecules to be used for energy. Only liver cells (hepatocytes) and muscle cells (myocytes) have the needed enzyme to complete this reaction. Only liver cells have the enzyme necessary to release glucose back into the bloodstream.

glycolysis A set of chemical reactions that generate energy from splitting glucose (a six-carbon molecule) into two pyruvate molecules (three carbons each). In the process, two "energy" molecules of adenosine triphosphate (ATP) are produced.

homeostasis In biology, the state or maintenance of balance or equilibrium.

hyperplasia When a tissue is enlarged due to replication or proliferation of cells.

hypertension A medical condition characterized by high blood pressure.

hypertrophy The increase in size or enlargement of a cell.

in vitro A process that takes place outside a biological environment (e.g., in a test tube or culture dish).

in vivo A process that takes place "in life" or within a living organism or cell.

inflammation A biological response to an injury or infection. Characterized by the five signs of heat, pain, redness, swelling, and loss of function (calor, dolor, rubor, tumor, and functio laesa). Can be acute or chronic, localized or systemic.

insulin-like growth factor 1 (IGF-1) A hormone-signaling molecule with anabolic (or growth) properties. Among other functions, IGF-1 has been identified to promote growth of cancer cells.

insulin resistance (IR) When cells do not respond to the insulin hormone.

intermittent fasting (IF) A type of eating pattern that cycles between periods of feeding (eating) and fasting, typically repeated on an ongoing daily or weekly basis. Includes time-restricted eating (TRE), alternate-day fasting (ADF), and twice-weekly fasting (TWF).

ketones (or ketone bodies) In organic chemistry, compounds that contain a specific structure known as a ketone group. In biology, the liver and kidneys can produce these compounds from fat breakdown, and they can be used as an alternative energy source when carbohydrates are not available.

ketosis The metabolic state in which the body is using fat for fuel. It is characterized by the increase in ketone measures in the blood or urine.

leptin A type of adipokine involved in regulation of energy expenditure through suppression of appetite and regulation of fat storage; has pro-inflammatory properties. Also known as the "satiety hormone."

life span The length of life of an organism or person.

lipid In chemistry, another term for fats, types of compounds that are not soluble in water.

lipogenesis The set of chemical reactions that create larger fat molecules from smaller fatty acids and glycerol for storage.

lipolysis *Lipo* means "fat" and *lysis* means "to break down." Lipolysis is the set of chemical reactions that break down fat into smaller molecules of free fatty acids and glycerol. Glycerol can be used in gluconeogenesis.

lipoproteins Molecules made up of protein and fat, which usually carry cholesterol and other fats through the bloodstream. Includes low-density lipoprotein (LDL), very low-density lipoprotein (VLDL), and high-density lipoprotein (HDL).

macronutrients Nutrients, including carbohydrates, fats, and protein, that are needed in large amounts for our cellular physiology to function normally.

maladaptive Not being able to adjust or adapt appropriately to changes in an environment.

meta-analysis A statistical analysis that combines data or findings from multiple independent studies.

metabolism A group of chemical reactions that are essential to maintaining cellular functions. The reactions either generate or use energy to create structures.

micelles Particles that tend to aggregate together in solution. In the body, *micelle* refers to fat particles grouping together in aqueous (watery) solution.

microbiome *Biome* refers to a community of biological organisms in a given environment; *micro* refers to microorganisms such as bacteria, fungi, or viruses. The gut microbiome is a community of organisms found inside the gut lining of the large intestine. There are other microbiomes in the body according to their anatomical location (e.g., skin, oral mucosa, vagina).

micronutrients Nutrients, such as vitamins and minerals, that are needed in small amounts from the diet but are essential for our cellular physiology to function normally.

minimally supplemented fasting A type of prolonged fast (PF) where 75 to 250 calories of juices and soups are consumed per day, typically for up to 21 days.

naturopathic An approach to medicine that seeks to achieve healing primarily through natural therapies, such as lifestyle modifications, nutrition, exercise, and the use of herbs.

noncommunicable disease Diseases that are not infectious or transmissible in nature and are typically long in duration, or chronic.

obesogens Chemical substances that are said to disrupt metabolism and may lead to the development of obesity.

pathological A disease state or abnormal functioning.

peptide A compound made of a chain of two or more amino acids.

physiological Relates to normal functioning or adaptations of the body.

polypharmacy The simultaneous use of multiple medications by a single patient to treat one or multiple conditions.

prolonged fasting (PF) Partial or total caloric restriction for a period of up to 40 days. Includes minimally supplemented fasting and water-only fasting.

prolonged water-only fasting Type of prolonged fast (PF) in which only water is consumed for up to 40 days, typically while under medical supervision. Also called zero-calorie fasting.

prospective study Type of scientific study that observes outcomes of a test group over a period of time.

randomized controlled trial Type of prospective study that compares an experimental group to a control group (group that has not gone under the experiment's design).

retrospective study Type of scientific study that uses data or information that was collected in the past.

SOS-free diet A type of diet comprised exclusively of whole-plant foods free of added salt, oil, and sugar; promoted by TrueNorth Health Center.

starvation Process characterized by a decline in fat metabolism and an increase in the synthesis of new glucose from recycled cellular material, including protein, in an environment of nutrient depletion.

steady-state When a process that was initiated is then maintained over time.

subcutaneous adipose tissue A component of total body fat found below the skin.

TCA cycle In biochemistry, a set of chemical reactions that occur inside the mitochondria of the cell in the presence of oxygen (cellular respiration) to produce energy. Also called tricarboxylic acid cycle, or citric acid cycle, or Krebs cycle.

temperance The practice of moderation or self-restraint.

therapeutic fasting A fasting process that is voluntarily applied for the purpose of healing.

time-restricted eating (TRE) A type of intermittent fasting (IF) that involves eating within a specified time period and abstaining from caloric intake (i.e., fasting) for the rest of the day.

twice-weekly fasting (TWF) A type of intermittent fasting (IF) that includes five days of unrestricted eating and two "fasting" days with significant caloric restriction; can follow a consecutive or nonconsecutive pattern. Also known as the 5:2 diet.

urea cycle Amino acids are nitrogen-containing compounds that can form ammonia. Ammonia is toxic, but the body has an impressive way of "clearing" ammonia by converting it to urea, a chemical compound that is not toxic and can be excreted. This happens through a series of chemical reactions known as the urea cycle.

visceral adipose tissue (VAT) A component of total body fat that is found around the abdominal organs (or viscera). It is metabolically active tissue that releases hormones.

SUSTAINED CHANGES IN CARDIOMETABOLIC BIOMARKERS AFTER FASTING

BIOMARKER		BL	EOF	EOR	FU
BW, lb		196.4	176.6	179.9	177.0
BMI, kg/m^2	(18.5–24.9 kg/m^2)	32.3	29.5	29.6	29.1
AC, in (women)	(<34.6 in)	39.5	35.8	37.0	36.8
AC, in (men)	(<40.1 in)	40.1	35.4	37.6	40.4
SBP, mmHg	(<120 mmHg)	123	113	110	114
DBP, mmHg	(<80 mmHg)	78	80	76	78
TC, mmol/L	(2.59–5.15 mmol/L)	5.1	5.06	4.65	4.61
LDL, mmol/L	(<2.56 mmol/L)	3.17	3.28	2.72	2.72
HDL, mmol/L	(>1.01 mmol/L)	1.29	1.15	1.14	1.19
VLDL, mmol/L	(0.13–1.04 mmol/L)	0.49	0.6	0.69	0.57
TAGs, mmol/L	(<3.86 mmol/L)	1.16	1.48	1.68	1.45
Glucose, mmol/L	(3.61–5.49 mmol/L)	5.19	4.38	5.47	5
Insulin, pmol/L	(15.6–149.4 pmol/L)	50	31	62	41
HOMA-IR	(<1.9 insulin sensitive)	1.85	1.04	2.56	1.51
GGT, nmol/(s*L)	(<1000 nmol/(s*L))	250	250	250	233
FLI	(<30 is optimal)	65	45	57	47
hsCRP, mg/L	(<3 mg/L)	1.83	2.63	1.06	0.9

Note: Labcorp reference ranges for normal values are provided beside the respective biomarker. *N* = 38 at BL, EOF, and EOR. *N* = 33 at FU. AC, abdominal circumference; BL, baseline; BMI, body mass index; BW, body weight; DBP, diastolic blood pressure; EOF, end of fast; EOR, end of refeeding; FLI, fatty liver index; FU, follow-up; GGT, gamma-glutamyl transferase; HDL, high-density lipoprotein; HOMA-IR, homeostatic model assessment of insulin resistance; hsCRP, high-sensitivity C-reactive protein; in, inches; kg, kilogram; lb, pounds; LDL, low-density lipoprotein; m, meter; mg/L, milligram per liter; mmHg, millimeters of mercury; mmol/L, millimole per liter; nmol/(s*L), nanomole per second liter; pmol/L, picomole per liter; SBP, systolic blood pressure; TAGs, triglycerides; TC, total cholesterol; VLDL, very low-density lipoprotein.

COMMON BIOMARKER RANGES, FUNCTIONS, AND INDICATIONS

BIOMARKER	AGE	REFERENCE RANGE	FUNCTION	DISEASE INDICATION
Total cholesterol	>19	100–199 mg/dL	Maintains integrity and fluidity of cell membranes. Helps build new tissue and repair damage to existing tissue. Produces steroid hormones, including estrogen. Helps create bile in the liver. Aids in production of vitamin D.	High levels associated with CVD.
Triglycerides	>19	0–149 mg/dL	Storage of energy.	
HDL cholesterol	>19	>39 mg/dL	Absorbs cholesterol and carries it back to the liver, where it is flushed out.	High levels can lower risk of CVD.
VLDL cholesterol	>19	5–40 mg/dL	Carries mostly triglycerides to tissues.	High levels can build up on the walls of blood vessels (plaque), which can lead to CVD.
LDL cholesterol	>19	0–99 mg/dL	Carries cholesterol to tissues.	High levels can build up on the walls of blood vessels (plaque), which can lead to CVD.
ApoB		<90 mg/dL	Acts as a ligand for LDL receptors for cholesterol uptake and LDL catabolism in various cell types of the body. Atherogenic lipoproteins (VLDL, IDL, LDL, and Lp(a)) contain a single ApoB protein.	More accurate measure of heart-disease risk. High levels can increase the risk of plaque (see VLDL, LDL).

BIOMARKER	AGE	REFERENCE RANGE	FUNCTION	DISEASE INDICATION
Glucose		65–99 mg/dL	Source of energy and essential to fuel both aerobic and anaerobic cellular respiration.	High fasting glucose (diabetes) is associated with CVD; nerve damage (neuropathy); kidney damage (diabetic nephropathy) or kidney failure; and damage to the blood vessels of the retina (diabetic retinopathy), which could lead to blindness.
hsCRP		0.00–3.00 mg/L	Binds to determinants on microorganisms and damaged cells; activates the classical complement pathway.	Marker of inflammation.
Insulin		2.6–24.9 ulU/mL	Regulates the body's energy supply by balancing micronutrient levels during the fed state. Critical for transporting intracellular glucose to insulin-dependent cells/tissues, such as liver, muscle, and adipose tissues.	High levels increase the risk of obesity, type 2 diabetes, and CVD and decreases health span and life expectancy.
GGT		Female: 0–60 IU/L Male: 0–65 IU/L	Helps move other molecules around the body; plays a significant role in helping the liver metabolize drugs and other toxins.	High levels in the blood may be a sign of liver disease and CVD.
IGF-1		Varies from 109 to 265 ng/GGT (median), depending on age, diet.	Major mediator of growth hormone-stimulated somatic growth as well as a mediator of growth hormone-independent anabolic responses in many cells and tissues.	High levels have been associated with risk of several types of cancer.

(continued)

BIOMARKER	AGE	REFERENCE RANGE	FUNCTION	DISEASE INDICATION
ANTHROPOMETRIC BIOMARKERS				
SBP/DBP		<120/<80 mmHg		
Waist circumference		Female: <88 cm Male: <102 cm		
BMI		18.5–24.99 kg/m^2		
MARKERS FOR METABOLIC HEALTH				
FLI		0–30		Based on waist circumference, BMI, triglyceride, and GGT for the prediction of fatty liver.
HOMA-IR		<1.9		Homeostatic model assessment of insulin resistance based on glucose and insulin levels.
GENERAL BIOMARKERS MONITORED DURING FASTING				
White blood cells		3.4–10.8 x10E3/uL		
Red blood cells		Female: 3.77–5.28 x10E6/uL Male: 4.14–5.8 x10E6/uL		
Hemoglobin		Female: 11.1–15.9 g/dL Male: 13.0–17.7 g/dL		
Hematocrit		Female: 34.0–46.6% Male: 37.5–51.0%		

BIOMARKER	AGE	REFERENCE RANGE	FUNCTION	DISEASE INDICATION
GENERAL BIOMARKERS MONITORED DURING FASTING *(continued)*				
MCV		79–97 fL		
MCH		26.6–33.0 pg		
MCHC		31.5–35.7 g/dL		
RDW		Female: 11.7–15.4% Male: 11.6–15.4%		
Platelets		150–450 x10E3/uL		
Neutrophils		1.4–7.0 x10E3/uL		
Lymphocytes		0.7–3.1 x10E3/uL		
Monocytes		0.1–0.9 x10E3/uL		
EOS		0.0–0.4 x10E3/uL		
Basophils		0.0–0.2 x10E3/uL		
Immature granulocytes		0.0–0.1 x10E3/uL		
BUN	18 to 59	Female: 9–23 Male: 9–20		
	>59	Female: 12–28 Male: 10–24		

(continued)

BIOMARKER	AGE	REFERENCE RANGE	FUNCTION	DISEASE INDICATION
GENERAL BIOMARKERS MONITORED DURING FASTING *(continued)*				
Creatinine	>14	Female: 0.57–1.00 mg/dL Male: 0.76–1.27 mg/dL		
Estimated glomerular filtration rate		>59 mL/min/1.73		
BUN/creatinine ratio	18 to 59	Female: 9–23 Male: 9–20		
	>59	Female: 12–28 Male: 10–24		
Sodium		134–144 mEq/L		
Potassium		3.5–5.2 mEq/L		
Chloride		96–106 mmol/L		
Carbon dioxide		20–29 mmol/L		
Calcium	18–59	8.7–10.2 mg/dL		
	>59	Female: 8.7–10.3 mg/dL Male: 8.6–10.2 mg/dL		
Protein		6.0–8.5 g/dL		
Albumin	31–50	Female: 3.8–4.8 g/dL Male: 4.0–5.0 g/dL		

BIOMARKER	AGE	REFERENCE RANGE	FUNCTION	DISEASE INDICATION
GENERAL BIOMARKERS MONITORED DURING FASTING *(continued)*				
	51–60	3.8–4.9 g/dL		
	61–70	3.8–4.8 g/dL		
	71–80	3.7–4.7 g/dL		
Globulin		1.5–4.5 g/dL		
A/G ratio		1.2–2.2		
Bilirubin		0.0–1.2 mg/dL		
Alkaline phosphatase		44–121 IU/L		
AST (SGOT)		0–40 IU/L		
ALT (SGPT)		Female: 0–32 IU/L Male: 0–44 IU/L		

Note: ALT (SGPT), alanine aminotransferase (serum glutamic-pyruvic transaminase); ApoB, apolipoprotein B; AST (SGOT), aspartate aminotransferase (serum glutamic-oxaloacetic transaminase); BUN, blood urea nitrogen; CMP, comprehensive metabolic panel; CVD, cardiovascular disease; EOS, eosinophil count; fL, femtoliter; g/dL, grams per deciliter; GGT, gamma-glutamyl transferase; hsCRP, high-sensitivity C-reactive protein; IU/L, international units per liter; Lp(a), lipoprotein (a); MCH, mean corpuscular hemoglobin; MCHC, mean corpuscular hemoglobin concentration; MCV, mean corpuscular volume; mEq/L, milliequivalents per liter; mg/dl, milligrams per deciliter; mL/min/1.73, milliliters per minute per 1.73; ng/mL, nanograms per milliliter; pg, picogram; RDW, red cell distribution width; uIU/ml, micro-international units per microliter; VLDL, very low-density lipoprotein; x10E3/uL, 10,000 per microliter; x10E6/uL, 1,000,000 per microliter.

APPENDIX 4

SUSTAINED CHANGES IN BLOOD PRESSURE AFTER FASTING

Changes in blood pressure by stage and visit

BASELINE (SBP/DBP, mmHg)		BL	EOF	EOR	6wFU	12mFU
All	SBP	147	117	113	122	125
	DBP	86	75	77	76	74
130 to 139/80 to 89 (stage 1)	SBP	135	112	111	118	127
	DBP	82	73	73	74	75
≥140/≥90 (stage 2)	SBP	158	121	115	125	122
	DBP	90	76	80	78	73

Table data source: TNHF unpublished data. Note: 6wFU, six-week follow-up; 12mFU, twelve-month follow-up; BL, baseline; DBP, diastolic blood pressure; EOF, end of fast; EOR, end of refeeding; mmHg, millimeters of mercury; SBP, systolic blood pressure.

INTERPRETING VITAL SIGNS AND LABS DURING FASTING

Vital signs

Body weight and BMI	Use caution with too rapid BW loss beyond what is known to occur during fasting (1–2 lbs/day): consider discontinuation of fasting when BMI drops below limit of normal (18.5%)
Body temperature	Despite colder extremities and decrease in BMR, there are no significant changes; warm clothes and blankets can help ease the fasting process
Pulse	Variations in pulse may be present; a manual pulse check is recommended to check for rhythm, rate, force, equality
Blood pressure	Decreases; use caution with activities that may lower BP such as hot showers, saunas, too much sun exposure
SpO2	No change

Changes in lab values during fasting

LAB	CHANGES DURING FASTED STATE	NOTES
CBC		
White blood cells	↓	Changes WNL; if increased suspect infection
Red blood cells	↑*	Changes WNL; may be due to hemoconcentration from dehydration
Hematocrit	↑*	Changes WNL; may be due to hemoconcentration from dehydration
Hemoglobin	↑*	Changes WNL; may be due to hemoconcentration from dehydration
MCV, MCH, MCHC, RDW, MPV	No change	Fluctuate WNL
Platelet count	No change	Fluctuate WNL
Neutrophils, lymphocytes, monocytes, eosinophils, basophils	No change	White blood cells break down; important only if white blood cells are high
Sedimentation rate	No change	Marker of inflammation; if greater than 90, explore an autoimmune diagnosis

(continued)

LAB	CHANGES DURING FASTED STATE	NOTES
CMP		
Glucose	↓*	Changes WNL; if low and symptomatic, break fast using vegetable juice
Sodium	↓*	Changes WNL; if low and symptomatic, reduce water intake if indicated or break fast using vegetable broth or juice
Potassium	↓*	Changes WNL; if low and symptomatic, break fast using vegetable broth or juice
Chloride	↓*	Changes WNL; may follow similar trend as sodium
Carbon dioxide	↓*	May be compensation due to increased acidity from ketones
BUN	↓	Changes WNL
BUN/creatinine	↓*	
Creatinine	↑*	Changes WNL; if significant increase, break fast
Calcium	No change	
Alkaline phosphate	No change	
Protein total	↑*	Changes WNL
Albumin	↑*	Changes WNL
Globulin	↑*	Changes WNL
A/G ratio	No change	May be relevant in the presence of severe liver disease
Bilirubin total	↑	Changes WNL
AST (SGOT)	↑*	Changes WNL
ALT (SGTP)	↑*	Changes WNL
Estimated glomerular filtration rate	↓*	Changes WNL; if significant decrease, break fast
Uric acid	↑	
LDH	↓	Changes a concern only if patient has liver disease

*During fasting, all return to normal limits upon refeeding.

Note: A/G, albumin/globulin; ALT, alanine transaminase; ALT (SGPT), alanine aminotransferase (serum glutamic-pyruvic transaminase); AST, aspartate aminotransferase; AST (SGOT), aspartate aminotransferase (serum glutamic-oxaloacetic transaminase); BMI, body mass index; BMR, basal metabolic rate; BP, blood pressure; BUN, blood urea nitrogen; BW, body weight; CBC, complete blood count; CMP, comprehensive metabolic panel; LDH, lactate dehydrogenase; MCH, mean corpuscular hemoglobin; MCHC, mean corpuscular hemoglobin concentration; MCV, mean corpuscular volume; MPV, mean platelet volume; RDW, red cell distribution width; SpO2, oxygen saturation; WNL, within normal limits.

PROLONGED WATER-ONLY FASTING SUPERVISION PROTOCOL CHECKLIST

Pre-fast

PREPARATION (AT LEAST TWO DAYS PRIOR)

- Eliminate all harmful substances (e.g., coffee, alcohol, nicotine)
- Eliminate grains, legumes, dairy, meat, sugar, oils, salt, and all processed foods
- Consume only raw fruits and vegetables and steamed vegetables

EXAMINATIONS

- Detailed patient history; ensure adequate evacuations and bowel movements before initiating fast
- Comprehensive physical exam, including height, weight, temperature, blood pressure, pulse
- Basic neurological and psychological status
- Complete blood count (CBC) with differential
- Comprehensive metabolic panel (CMP)
- Urine analysis (UA)
- Additional tests as clinically indicated

MEDICATIONS AND SUPPLEMENTS

- Taper off all medications that can be safely discontinued
- Hormone replacement medications can be continued at reduced dosage
- Taper off and discontinue all supplements
- If medications cannot be discontinued, alternative treatment is indicated

Fast

THERAPY

- Steam-distilled water (minimum 40 oz/day)
- Limit excessive physical activity
- Rest and relaxation
- Termination: by patient request or when medically necessary

EXAMINATIONS

- Vital signs (2x/day)
- General symptom inquiry (2x/day): monitor for known side effects of fasting such as emerging nausea, headaches, lightheadedness, changes in sleep patterns
- CBC, CMP, UA (1x/week)
- Additional tests as clinically indicated (as needed)
- Note: Bowel movements are uncommon during fasting; take note of last bowel movement or any emerging bowel movements

Post-fast

STANDARD REFEEDING*

- Duration is half of the fast's length
- Advise patient to chew food thoroughly
- One day on each phase for every 7 to 10 days of water-only fasting

PHASE 1: Fruit and vegetable juice (4x/day)

PHASE 2: Raw fruits (except citrus and pineapple) and raw juicy vegetables (3x/day)

PHASE 3: Raw fruits and vegetables, steamed vegetables (3x/day)

PHASE 4: Raw fruits and vegetables, steamed vegetables, grains, soups, and nuts (up to 1 oz/day) or avocado (half/day) (3x/day)

PHASE 5: Unrestricted plant-food diet free of added sugar, oil, and salt (3x/day)

*Sensitive refeeding plans exclude foods known to cause inflammation in patient

EXAMINATIONS

- Continue monitoring of vital signs and making general symptom inquiry (2x/day)
- Labs during this phase are not necessary but may be performed as clinically indicated

MISCELLANEOUS

- Bowel movements begin gradually over course of refeeding
- May slowly increase physical activity

APPENDIX 7

STEPWISE REFEEDING DIET

TrueNorth Health Center Standard Refeeding Guidelines

PHASE 1: JUICE		
1 day juicing for every 7 to 10 days of fasting	Four juices/day If the first juices taste too strong, please dilute them with water, and do drink them all down	
PHASE 2: RAW		
1 day raw for every 7 to 10 days of fasting	Raw fruits (except citrus and pineapple) Raw, juicy vegetables (e.g., lettuce, cucumber, tomato, celery, jicama, sprouts)	
PHASE 3: STEAMED		
1 day of raw and steamed plants for every 7 to 10 days of fasting	Raw fruits Steamed vegetables Light soups (without grains)	Potatoes, yams, squash Premade, grain-free salads Dressings (small amounts)
PHASE 4: GRAINS, NUTS AND SEEDS, AND AVOCADO		
1–2 days of raw and steamed plants and grains for every 7 to 10 days of fasting	Raw fruits Raw vegetables Premade salads and all cold foods Grains (oatmeal, rice, quinoa, corn)	Steamed vegetables Avocado (up to half per day) Nuts or seeds (½ oz) *No legumes*
PHASE 5: UNRESTRICTED		
SOS-free diet indefinitely	Raw fruits Raw vegetables Premade salads and all cold foods Grains (oatmeal, rice, quinoa, corn) Nuts and seeds (up to 1 oz per day)	Steamed vegetables Avocado (up to half per day) Thick soups Legumes Prepared desserts

APPENDIX 8

RESOURCES

Medically Supervised Water-Only Fasting Facilities

TrueNorth Health Center and Phone Coaching Services
healthpromoting.com

Clinical Training in Prolonged Water-Only Fasting Supervision

TrueNorth Health Center
healthpromoting.com

Research and Education

TrueNorth Health Foundation
fasting.org

SOS-Free Diet Resources

First Seed
firstseedfoods.com/collections/frontpage
Enter code TrueNorth at checkout for $10 off your purchase.

LeafSide
goleafside.com/truenorth

National Health Association
healthscience.org

Straight Up Food
straightupfood.com/blog

Well Your World
wellyourworld.com/truenorth

Whole Harvest
wholeharvest.com/truenorth

INDEX

Please note that the letter f appearing immediately after a page number refers to a figure on that page; the letter t refers to a table on that page.

C

S

U

V

Y

Z

ABOUT THE AUTHORS

Toshia Myers, PhD, is the director of the TrueNorth Health Foundation. Dr. Myers's scientific curiosity was first piqued by the intricacies of cellular biology as an undergraduate at The Ohio State University. Later, she completed a doctorate of philosophy in biological sciences at Columbia University, specializing in molecular genetics and developmental biology. She then completed postdoctoral fellowships at the Centers for Disease Control and Prevention and the University of Copenhagen Biotech Research and Innovation Centre, where she focused on immunology and epigenetics. While in graduate school, she was struck by the profound implications of natural hygiene and the ability of these basic principles to improve and maintain her own health, which led her to combine her passion for research and natural health. At the TrueNorth Health Foundation, she oversees clinical research into the effects of prolonged water-only fasting on human health.

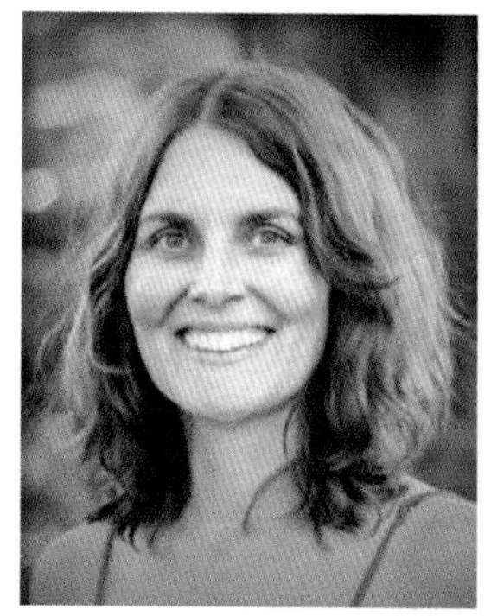

Dr. Alan Goldhamer is an expert in the use of medically supervised water-only fasting. He is the founder and has been the director of TrueNorth Health Center since 1984 and has supervised the fasting and care of more than 25,000 patients. TrueNorth Health Center is a multidisciplinary practice that includes doctors of medicine, osteopathy, chiropractic, naturopathy, and psychology. The center's healthcare providers treat patients with conditions ranging from high blood pressure and diabetes to autoimmune disorders and lymphoma. It is the largest facility in the world specializing in medically supervised water-only fasting and is a premier training facility for doctors to gain certification in the supervision of therapeutic fasting.

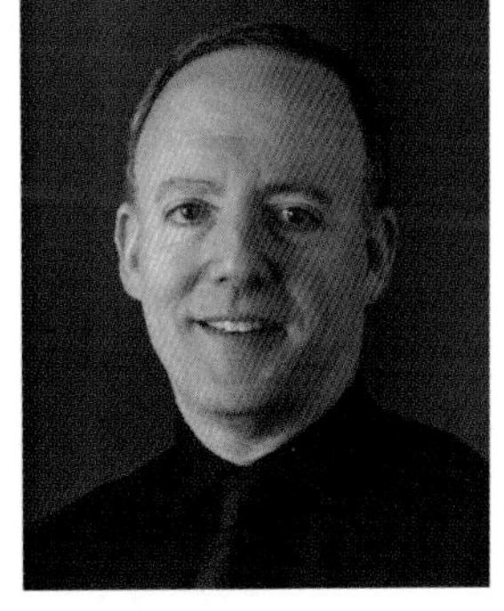

Dr. Goldhamer is the author of *The Health Promoting Cookbook* and coauthor of *The Pleasure Trap: Mastering the Hidden Force That Undermines Health and Happiness*. He has helped author numerous studies and case reports published in peer-reviewed journals. He is a frequent lecturer, speaking on the use of fasting and diet in the restoration of optimal health.

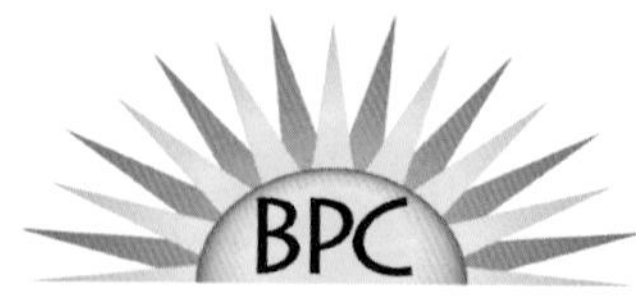

books that educate, inspire, and empower

To find your favorite books on plant-based cooking and nutrition, natural wellness solutions, and sustainable living, visit **bookpubco.com.**

More titles from Alan Goldhamer and TrueNorth Health Center

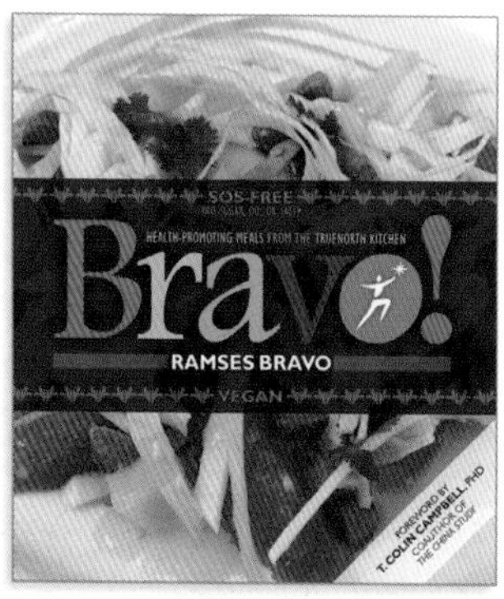

Bravo!
Health Promoting Recipes
from the TrueNorth Health Kitchen
Ramses Bravo
$24.95 • 978-1-57067-269-9

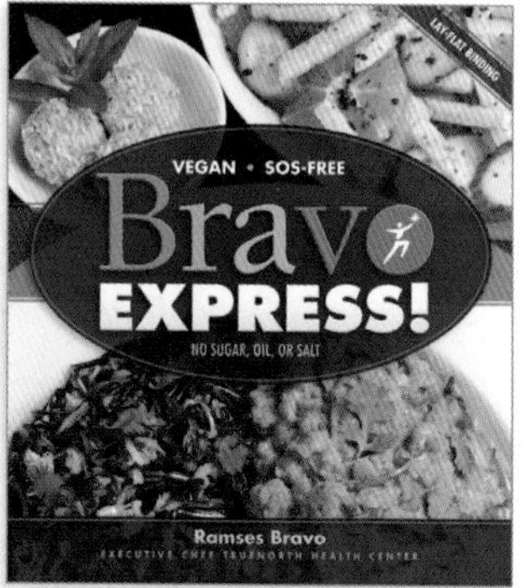

Bravo Express!
Ramses Bravo
$24.95 • 978-1-57067-362-7

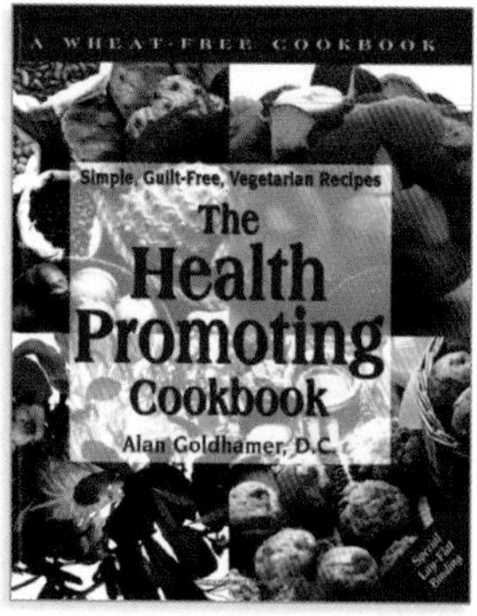

The Health Promoting Cookbook
Simple, Guilt-Free Vegetarian Recipes
Alan Goldhamer, DC
$16.95 • 978-1-57067-024-4

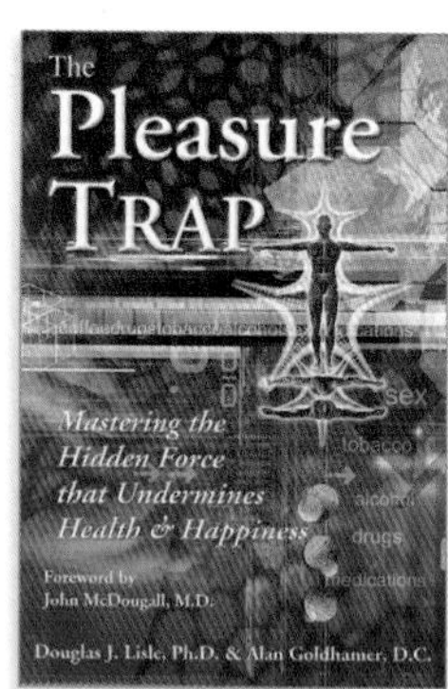

The Pleasure Trap
Mastering the Hidden Force that
Undermines Health & Happiness
Douglas J. Lisle, PhD, and Alan Goldhamer, DC
$19.95 • 978-1-57067-197-5

Purchase these titles from your favorite book source or buy them directly from
BPC • PO Box 99 • Summertown, TN 38483 • 1-888-260-8458

Free shipping and handling on all orders